Hair Cells and Hearing Aids

Hair Cells and Hearing Aids

Edited by Charles I. Berlin, Ph.D.
Kresge Hearing Research Laboratory of the South
Department of Otolaryngology and Biocommunication
Louisiana State University Medical Center
New Orleans, Louisiana

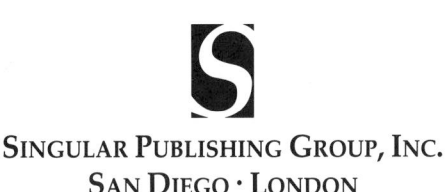

SINGULAR PUBLISHING GROUP, INC.
SAN DIEGO · LONDON

Singular Publishing Group, Inc.
4284 41st Street
San Diego, California 92105-1197

19 Compton Terrace
London, N1 2UN

©1996 by Singular Publishing Group, Inc.

Typeset in 10/12 Palatino by So Cal Graphics
Printed in the United States of America by McNaughton and Gunn

All rights, including that of translation, reserved. No part of this publication may be reproduced, stored in a retrieval system, or transmitted in any form or by any means, electronic, mechanical, recording, or otherwise, without the prior written permission of the publisher.

Library of Congress Cataloging-in-Publication Data

Hair cells and hearing aids/ [edited by] Charles I. Berlin.
    p.   cm.
  Based on a symposium.
  ISBN 1-56593-403-2
  1. Hair cells. 2. Hearing aids—Fitting. 3. Otoacoustic emissions.
I. Berlin, Charles I.
RF300.H34 1995
617.8'9—dc20   95–34353
                                                                             CIP

Contents

Preface   vii

A Brief History of the Laboratory   ix

1: Outer Hair Cell Electromotility and Otoacoustic Emissions   3
William E. Brownell, Ph.D.

2: Chemical Receptors on Outer Hair Cells and Their Molecular Mechanisms   29
Richard P. Bobbin, Ph.D.

3: Suppression of Otoacoustic Emissions in Normal Hearing Individuals   57
Linda J. Hood, Ph.D., Charles I. Berlin, Ph.D., Annette Hurley, M.S., and Han Wen, M.S.B.M.E.

4: Cochlear Outer Hair Cells vis-á-vis Semicircular Canal Type II Hair Cells   73
Charles H. Norris, Ph.D.

5: Genetics and Hair Cell Loss   87
Bronya J. B. Keats, Ph.D., Nassim Nouri, M.S., Jer-Min Huang, M.D., Ph.D., Matthew Money, M.D., Douglas B. Webster, Ph.D., Mary Z. Pelias, Ph.D., and Charles I. Berlin, Ph.D.

6: Hearing Aids: Only for Hearing-Impaired Patients with Abnormal Otoacoustic Emissions   99
Charles I. Berlin, Ph.D., Linda J. Hood, Ph.D., Annette Hurley, M.S., and Han Wen, M.S.B.M.E.

7: Multichannel Compression in Hearing Aids   113
Edgar Villchur

8: Talking Hair Cells: What They Have to Say About Hearing Aids   125
Mead C. Killion, Ph.D.

Index   x

Preface

Most people who have hearing losses have been told in the past that they have "nerve deafness." We can now distinguish between nerve deafness and hair cell deafness in a manner that affects what types of hearing aids we fit to patients and how. This symposium brings together world renowned scientists to show us how and why we can improve our patient care and management.

We have assembled summaries of our current understanding of the relationships of hair cell micromechanics, chemistry, genetics, and otoacoustic emissions to hearing aid fitting. Coupled to the 25th Anniversary celebration of the Kresge Hearing Research Laboratory of the South, at Louisiana State University Medical School's Department of Otolaryngology and Biocommunication, this compilation shows the close relationship of basic science to clinical care which has been the hallmark of our organization.

Brownell's work shows the nature of the electromotility he discovered. This was the missing concept in understanding how and why the ear could respond to such faint levels of input, without violating laws of physics which predicted a cochlear displacement at "threshold" that was inconceivably small.

Bobbin and Norris show the electrochemical and related factors that contribute to hair cell motility in the auditory versus vestibular systems, while Keats tells us of the genetic nature of hair cell loss and her group's discovery of a gene for recessive deafness and hair cell loss on chromosome 19 of the *dn/dn* mouse.

Hood reviews the work on one of the acoustic products of hair cell motility, the otoacoustic emission, and how this emission can be used as a noninvasive acoustic microscope, addressing the integrity of outer hair cell systems. Berlin shows how the efferent system suppresses outer hair cell motility in the presence of noise in either or both ears, and how, in some patients whose audiograms may indicate serious hearing loss, normal otoacoustic emissions preclude the use of hearing aids. He also discusses a model of recruitment and hearing aid fitting that sets the stage for the final two chapters on hearing aids.

Villchur and Killion conclude the symposium with the rationales and mechanisms behind their hearing aid design principles; these remarkable developments led to the ReSound and K-Amp aids and all their descendants. These hearing aids help us manage hair cell sensory loss at a level of success heretofore impossible by mimicking the missing high gain functions of outer hair cells only at low intensities. The gain of the aids becomes either transparent or compressed at high intensity inputs, thus compensating to a great extent for recruitment of loudness.

In summary, this symposium takes us from important discoveries about the nature of the inner ear, how they manifest themselves clinically, and how we can use these discoveries and principles to improve the quality of life of our patients who have sensory hearing losses.

A Brief History of the Laboratory

The Laboratory owes its existence to the vision and determination of Irving Blatt, M.D. It was he who brought me down to New Orleans in June of 1967 to start what was then called the Communication Sciences Laboratory (CSL). Dr. Blatt, who was a graduate of the University of Michigan's residency program, had been impressed with the Kresge Hearing Research Institute at Michigan, which was started by Merle Lawrence, Ph.D., in 1950. Blatt wanted a similar research program in his department and, soon after we started the CSL lab, he urged me to write to the Kresge Foundation in Michigan for support.

The Kresge Foundation awarded us $100,000 to renovate a second of three buildings (Numbers 147, 148, and 164) that we ultimately occupied on the Florida Avenue (Dental School) Campus from 1967 to 1981. Soon after the Kresge Lab renovation was begun in 1970, Dr. Blatt left for private practice and Dr. George D. Lyons, Jr., became Head of the Otolaryngology Department. Then, in late 1981 and early 1982 we were moved from the barracks to a somewhat more livable structure on the same campus (Building 124) but were still separated from our parent Department of Otolaryngology and Biocommunication. We ultimately arrived in our current quarters on the first floor of 2020 Gravier St. in October of 1986.

Among the earliest personnel in the laboratory were Sena Lowe-Bell, Ph.D., Carl Thompson, Ph.D., Harriet Berlin, Gail Leslie, Deborah Majeau, M.D., Ph.D., John K. Cullen, Jr., Ph.D. (who was to serve as assistant director of the laboratory for years after he received his doctorate in 1975 from LSU's Department of Physiology), J.S. Soileau, M.D., Ray J. Lousteau, M.D., M.S. Ellis, M.D., and our first office manager, Gae O. Decker, whose staff included Wanda Bolleter and Ruth Goliwas. Subsequent office managers were Nancie Roark, Cindy Frazier, and Sue Northcutt. We are now ably managed by a crew of associates led by Judith Hull.

Drs. Larry Hughes, Doug Webster, and Richard Bobbin were on board by 1973, and Drs. Robert Porter, Terry Riemer, and Jim May held courtesy joint appointments through UNO. Dr. Linda Hood (1982), currently director of our Cochlear Implant Program, and Dr. Charles Parkins (1989) are our two latest full-time laboratory faculty appointments.

Dr. Bronya Keats, of the Department of Biometry and Genetics, is our latest and most welcome adjunct professor. Additional joint appointments included Drs. Paul Guth and Charles Norris from Tulane, Drs. Ray Daniloff, Paul Hoffman, Hugh Buckingham, Mick Miller, and Jane Collins from LSU in Baton Rouge, and Dr. Emily Tobey now of the Callier Center in Dallas. Faculty and post-doctoral fellows who have moved to other distinguished positions include: Michael Gorga, Ph.D., Pat Stelmachowicz, Ph.D., Glenis Long, Ph.D., Robert Dobie, M.D., Gary Jenison, M.D., Ph.D., David Chihal, M.D., Ph.D., Daniel Mouney, M.D., Linda Hood, Ph.D., Wayne Briner, Ph.D., Georgia Bryant, Ph.D., Sharon Kujawa, Ph.D., Ray Hurley, Ph.D., Phil McCandless Ph.D., and other colleagues and distinguished collaborators including Bill Sewell, Ph.D., Sandie Bledsoe, Ph.D., Jean Luc Puel, Ph.D., among others.

Key professional associates who worked at the laboratory included Joel Chatelain, Charles Wiesendanger, Anthony Florez, Prudence Allen, Peggy Pollack, Dorothea Morgan, Deirdre Rafferty, Ilene Rafferty, Elliot Smith, Robin Morehouse, Beth Barlow, Donna Ryan, M.D., Joseph Ryan, M.D., Pal Szabo, Dip. Eng., Steve Benton, Peggy Adams Noonan, Annette Hurley, and Drs. Li Li and Jer Min Huang, and Sam Abolrous and Han Wen, our computer and engineering specialists, respectively.

At our request, John K. Cullen Jr. prepared a lengthy and much more detailed history of the laboratory which is available on request.

Charles I. Berlin, Ph.D.
New Orleans, October 1995

Acknowledgments: NIDCD Center Grant P0 1 DC-000379, Training Grants T32-DC-00007, Department of Defense Neuroscience Center Grant via N. Bazan, Kam's Fund for Hearing Research, The Kleberg Foundation, Lions' Eye Foundation and District 8-S Charities. Special support for the entire document and this chapter as well came from Dr. S. Singh, Etymotic Research, Dr. A. Lippa and Hearing Innovations, and NDIB-BMDR 1549.

Contributors

Mead C. Killion, Ph.D.
Etymotics
Elk Grove Village, Illinois

Richard P. Bobbin, Ph.D.
Kresge Hearing Research Laboratory
LSU Medical Center
New Orleans, Louisiana

Linda J. Hood, Ph.D.
Kresge Hearing Research Laboratory
LSU Medical Center
New Orleans, Louisiana

Annette Hurley, M.S.
Kresge Hearing Research Laboratory
LSU Medical Center
New Orleans, Louisiana

Han Wen, M.S.B.E.
Kresge Hearing Research Laboratory
LSU Medical Center
New Orleans, Louisiana

Charles H. Norris, Ph.D.
Tulane University School of Medicine
New Orleans, Louisiana

Bronya J. B. Keats, Ph.D.
Molecular and Human Genetics Center
Kresge Hearing Research Laboratory
LSU Medical Center
New Orleans, Louisiana

Douglas B. Webster, Ph.D.
Kresge Hearing Research Laboratory
LSU Medical Center
New Orleans, Louisiana

Nassim Nouri, Ph.D.
Molecular and Human
Genetics Center
LSU Medical Center
New Orleans, Louisiana

Jer-Min Huang, M.D.
Kresge Hearing Research Laboratory
LSU Medical Center
New Orleans, Louisiana

Matthew Money, M.D.
Kresge Hearing Research Laboratory
LSU Medical Center
New Orleans, Louisiana

Mary Z. Pelias, Ph.D.
Molecular and Human
Genetics Center
LSU Medical Center
New Orleans, Louisiana

Edgar Villchur, President
Foundation for Hearing Research
Woodstock, New York

Introduction to Chapter 1

When Dr. Brownell accepted the First Kresge/Mirmelstein Award, he was in transition from the Johns Hopkins Medical Institutions to Baylor College of Medicine. In addition to a sterling recount of his original discovery and later observations, he presented a video tape of hair cells "dancing" to high amplitude electrical pulses transduced from a performance by rap artist MC Hammer. The transduction and video taping were done by a mutual colleague, Dr. Joseph Santos-Sacchi, and provided a stimulating and informative highlight of the presentation.

As part of his presentation, he introduced the analogy of the outer hair cells working in phase electrically with initial mechanical displacements, much the way a child "pumps" on a swing in synchrony with the direction and phase of displacement.

Time and circumstance did not permit a transcription of Brownell's exciting talk, but its high quality set the stage for the rest of the day. We are pleased to reprint here, with permission of the publishers, Dr. Brownell's germinal article on hair cell motility which appeared in the journal *Ear and Hearing* (Vol. 11, No. 2, 1990) and formed the basic data for the keynote address of this special occasion. Dr. Susan Jerger, Editor of the Journal, was instrumental in acquiring the permission.

Outer Hair Cell Electromotility and Otoacoustic Emissions

William E. Brownell
Department of Otolaryngology—Head and Neck Surgery,
Department of Neuroscience, and the Center for Hearing Sciences,
The Johns Hopkins University School of Medicine,
Baltimore, Maryland

Outer hair cell electromotility is a rapid, force generating, length change in response to electrical stimulation. DC electrical pulses either elongate or shorten the cell and sinusoidal electrical stimulation results in mechanical oscillations at acoustic frequencies. The mechanism underlying outer hair cell electromotility is thought to be the origin of spontaneous otoacoustic emissions. The ability of the cell to change its length requires that it be mechanically flexible. At the same time the structural integrity of the organ of Corti requires that the cell possess considerable compressive rigidity along its major axis. Evolution appears to have arrived at novel solutions to the mechanical requirements imposed on the outer hair cell. Segregation of cytoskeletal elements in specific intracellular domains facilitates the rapid movements. Compressive strength is provided by a unique hydraulic skeleton in which a positive hydrostatic pressure in the cytoplasm stabilizes a flexible elastic cortex with circumferential tensile strength. Cell turgor is required in order that the pressure gradients associated with the electromotile response can be communicated to the ends of the cell. A loss in turgor leads to loss of outer hair cell electromotility. Concentrations of salicylate equivalent to those that abolish spontaneous otoacoustic emissions in patients weaken the outer hair cell's hydraulic skeleton. There is a significant diminution in the electromotile response associated with the loss in cell turgor. Aspirin's effect on outer hair cell electromotility attests to the

> role of the outer hair cell in generating otoacoustic emissions and demonstrates how their physiology can influence the propagation of otoacoustic emissions.

There has been a dramatic change in our understanding of the biophysics of the mammalian inner ear over the past decade. The concept of the cochlea as a passive organ that converts the mechanical vibrations of sound into neural energy has been altered by the startling finding that outer hair cells possess a unique electromotile capacity (Brownell, 1983; 1984; Brownell, Bader, Bertrand, & de Ribaupierre, 1985). The electromotility appears to be responsible for the cochlea's surprising ability to generate sound (Kemp, 1978; see also other articles in this issue). The hearing science community now accepts the presence of otoacoustic emissions after nearly a decade of experimental confirmation. Skepticism from the more general sensory science community is understandable. The fact that the ear can make sound is, at one level, equivalent to the eye producing light or the nose expelling odors. Energy conversion in both directions (bidirectional transduction) appears unique to hearing and is thought to contribute to the remarkable sensitivity and exquisite frequency selectivity of mammalian hearing. This contribution is discussed below in a brief review of the evidence implicating outer hair cells in generating otoacoustic emissions. The physiological characteristics of outer hair cell electromotility is then presented followed by an analysis of the structure-function relationships within the organ of Corti. This analysis introduces the concept of the hydraulic skeleton as a solution for the mechanical requirements imposed on the outer hair cell. Evidence, including the effect of aspirin on outer hair cell turgor and its impact on otoacoustic emissions, is reviewed. The evidence supports the presence of a hydraulic skeleton.

EVIDENCE FOR A SOURCE OF MECHANICAL ENERGY IN THE COCHLEA

Investigations of the inner ear have, for years, been dominated by paradigms originally proposed by Helmholtz and implemented by Békésy. Békésy (1960) provided strong experimental evidence that the basilar membrane is mechanically tuned by demonstrating that it is most sensitive to low frequencies at one end of the cochlear spiral and high frequencies at the other. The accuracy and the functional importance of Békésy's findings stimulated inner ear research for decades.

The mechanical tuning Békésy measured was considerably broader than the neural tuning recorded from VIIIth nerve (Kiang, Watanabe, Thomas, & Clark, 1965) and the inner hair cell (Russell & Sellick, 1978). As new techniques were applied to the measurement of cochlear partition movement, each improvement resulted in narrower mechanical tuning curves and better agreement between mechanical and neural data (Khanna & Leonard, 1982; Rhode, 1971; Rhode, 1978; Robles, Ruggero, & Rich, 1986; Sellick, Patuzzi, & Johnstone, 1982). Anoxia or other insults to the cochlea lead to a degradation of the narrow mechanical tuning of a healthy ear till the movements resemble those measured by Békésy (Rhode, 1971; Sellick et al, 1982). These observations lead to the conclusion that narrow mechanical tuning of the living cochlea is based on a physiologically vulnerable mechanism. The change that follows anoxia and death suggests that an energy consuming or active process is required for normal tuning.

Békésy's description of the traveling wave motivated a number of mechanical engineering treatments. Analytic and numerical models were developed based on fundamental hydrodynamic and mechanical principles using passive mechanical elements. These models explain the general features of Békésy's traveling wave but they are unable to account for the narrow mechanical tuning measured in undamaged, living cochlea. Gold (1948) had made an early suggestion that mechanical energy from an active process in the cochlea could produce narrower mechanical tuning. Recent models (Geisler, 1986; Jen & Steele, 1987; Mountain, 1986; Neely & Kim, 1983), incorporating a source of mechanical energy and specifically electromechanical transduction in the cochlear partition, describe mechanical behavior that resembles the narrow tuning of the intact cochlea. The discovery (Kemp, 1978) and subsequent characterization of otoacoustic emissions (more fully described in other articles in this issue) supported the existence of the postulated source of mechanical energy in the cochlea. The evidence for sound production by the inner ear has been around for centuries. The annals of medicine provide numerous reports of sound coming from patients ears. While some of these sounds are noncochlear in origin, the possibility a cochlear origin for the remainder was not entertained until Kemp's demonstration of otoacoustic emissions in 1978.

EVIDENCE FOR AN OUTER HAIR CELL INVOLVEMENT IN OTOACOUSTIC EMISSIONS

The crossed olivo-cochlear bundle is a collection of neural fibers that originates in the brain stem and travels to the cochlea, terminating predominately on outer hair cells. Crossed olivo-cochlear bundle stimulation modulates inner hair cell receptor potentials without significantly changing their membrane resistance (Brown & Nuttal, 1984; Brown, Nuttal, & Masta, 1983). Such stimulation also changes the strength of acoustical distortion products in the ear canal (Mountain, 1980; Siegel & Kim, 1982). Both effects suggest an outer hair cell involvement in cochlear mechanics and specifically in the generation of otoacoustic emissions.

An outer hair cell involvement is also suggested by comparing the otoacoustic emissions produced by mammals and nonmammals. Otoacoustic emissions have been measured in vertebrates other than mammals (Klinke & Smolder, 1984; Manley & Schulze, 1987; Palmer & Wilson, 1981; Strack, KIinke, & Wilson, 1981; Whitehead, Wilson, & Baker, 1986; Wit, van Dijk, & Segenhaut, 1988) and are generally of lower magnitude and frequency than can be found in mammals. The hearing organs of most nonmammals bear a strong resemblance to the sensory epithelium of vertebrate vestibular organs. The bird's acoustic papilla has a dual hair cell organization (tall and short hair cells) with all the hair cells surrounded by supporting cells. Stimulated otoacoustic emissions, but not spontaneous otoacoustic emissions have been reported for the avian ear. The generation of otoacoustic emissions in nonmammalian species may result from electrically evoked movements of the stereociliar bundle (Assad, Hacohen, & Corey, 1989; Crawford & Fettiplace, 1985). Stereociliar bundle movements are low frequency events (<1 kHz) that match the otoacoustic emission frequencies measured in nonmammals. Mammalian otoacoustic emissions can occur at frequencies nearly an order of magnitude higher compelling us to look for structural features unique to the mammalian inner ear. The organ of Corti is a mammalian specialization and it was the discovery of the outer hair cell's unique electromotile response (Brownell, 1983; Brownell, 1984; Brownell et al, 1985) that greatly strengthened the possible role of the outer hair cell in generating otoacoustic emissions.

OUTER HAIR CELL ELECTROMOTILITY

Static Mechanical Features

The electromechanical abilities of the outer hair cell have been examined in isolated cells that have been dissociated from the organ of Corti and maintained with primary tissue culture techniques. Outer hair cells have proven tolerant of the procedures and have been maintained for up to 4 days (Brownell, 1983; Brownell, 1984; Brownell et al, 1985). The static mechanical features of the isolated cell provide the first hint of the cell's unique physiological characteristics. The healthy cell behaves as if it is a turgid rod. It resists bending and its cytoplasmic membranes resist deformation by probes. Evidence that the turgidity is related to a positive hydrostatic pressure comes from the fact that insults to the cytoplasmic membrane cause the cytoplasm to spew from the cell, often with sufficient force to eject the nucleus (Brownell, 1983; Brownell, 1984).

Shape Changes—Cell Length Increases or Decreases

Electrical stimulation of isolated outer hair cells generates reversible shape changes (Ashmore & Brownell, 1986; Brownell, 1983, 1984, 1986; Brownell et al, 1985; Brownell & Kachar, 1986; Evans, Dallos, & Hallworth, 1989; Holley & Ashmore, 1988a; Kachar, Brownell, Altschuler, & Fex, 1986; Santos-Sacchi, 1989; Santos-Sacchi & Dilger, 1988; Zenner, Zimmerman, & Schmitt, 1985). Length changes are the most conspicuous feature of the shape change because of the cell's cylindrical form. The cells elongate or shorten about a "resting length." The mechanism responsible for deforming the cell generates mechanical forces in opposite directions depending on the polarity of the electrical stimulus. While the force that is generated has not been directly measured, a single cell is able to move groups of attached cells that are many times its own mass. The ability of the outer hair cell to produce forces in opposite directions is the first of several physiological characteristics that distinguish outer hair cell electromotility from muscle cell motility. Skeletal muscle cells can generate force only when contracting. The relaxation phase of a skeletal muscle cell does not produce a force. Elongation of muscle cells is passive and generally occurs when forces produced by antagonistic muscles stretch the cell. The outer hair cell must either possess two carefully balanced mechanisms (of opposite sign) for producing its movements, or the movements are due to a single mechanism capable of producing force in either direction in response to electrical signals of opposite sign.

Voltage Dependence, Calcium Independence

The source of energy for outer hair cell electromotility appears to be the potential gradient that drives it. Partial evidence for this comes from experiments that demonstrate the movements are proportional to the applied voltage and not the current (Santos-Sacchi & Dilger, 1988). The movements occur even when most of the membrane ion channels have been blocked or if no calcium is present in the cell. The dependence on stimulus voltage and not stimulus current highlights yet another major difference between outer hair cell electromotility and conventional muscle motility.

Movements do not Require Cellular Stores of ATP

Further evidence that the movements result from a direct conversion of electrical potential energy to mechanical energy comes from experiments that demonstrate movements even after cellular stores of adenosine triphosphate (ATP) are depleted (Brownell & Kachar, 1986; Holley & Ashmore, 1988a; Kachar, Brownell, Altschuler & Fex, 1986). Muscle cells must convert cellular chemical energy stores in order to produce movements. They utilize a series of enzymatically driven biochemical steps that are triggered by an influx of calcium into the cell. The ATP independence of the outer hair cell movements is consistent with an absence of Na^+, K^+-ATPase in the outer hair cells (Drescher & Kerr, 1985; Kerr, Ross, & Ernst, 1982; Schulte & Adams, 1989). The absence of this enzyme is another unique feature of the outer hair cell. Na^+, K^+-ATPase is ubiquitous in animal cells and is generally essential for life as it helps to maintain transmembrane ionic gradients in the presence of leakage currents.

The outer hair cells have a number of different potassium channels (Ashmore & Meech, 1986; Gitter, Zenner, & Fromter, 1986; Santos-Sacchi & Dilger, 1988) and a portion of these channels are open at any one time. Outer hair cells will therefore begin to lose, and not be able to replenish intracellular potassium from the moment they are removed from the organ of Corti. The transmembrane concentration gradient for potassium will decline with the passage of time. The resting membrane potential will decline with the transmembrane concentration gradient. It is not surprising that their resting membrane potentials are low when measured in vitro with micropipettes (Brownell, 1983; Brownell, 1984; Brownell et al, 1985). When "patch" electrodes are used, the potassium inside the recording pipette quickly restores a "normal" potassium level to the cell and the resting membrane potential will generally stabilize near the high values (Gitter et al., 1986; Santos-Sacchi & Dilger, 1988) that have been measured in vivo (Dallos, Santos-Sacchi & Flock, 1982; Russell & Sellick, 1983). Outer hair cells maintain high "resting" membrane potentials in the intact cochlea even though they lack Na^+, K^+-ATPase because their intracellular potassium ion concentration is maintained by a standing current driven by the stria vascularis. A standing concentration gradient for potassium has been measured in scala tympani (Dulguerov, Zidanic, & Brownell, 1985; Johnstone, Patuzzi, Syka, & Sykova, 1989) which indicates that a significant portion of the standing current (silent current) is carried by potassium ions. The presence of the standing current was predicted by the high potassium ion concentration and the endocochlear potential found in scala media (Brownell, 1982; Brownell et al, 1986).

The Silent Current

The energy for muscle cell motility comes from cellular stores of adenosine triphosphate (ATP) produced in the cell via the Krebs cycle. Outer hair cell electromotility is also fueled by the Krebs cycle but the oxidative phosphorylation occurs outside the cell in a separate organ. ATP produced in the stria vascularis is used to drive an electrogenic pump in the marginal cells of that organ. In contrast to the outer hair cells, Na^+,K^+-ATPase is found throughout the stria vascularis and spiral ligament. These pumps give rise to the silent current illustrated in Figure 1–1 (Brownell, 1982; Brownell, Manis, Zidanic, & Spirou, 1983; Brownell, Zidanic, & Spirou, 1986; Zidanic & Brownell, 1989; Zidanic & Brownell, 1990). The receptor potential in the outer hair cell results from the modulation of the silent current. Outer hair cell electromotility is thought to be driven by the receptor potential, so that ultimately, the energy for the movements comes from the stria vascularis. The energy for movements observed in vitro derives from the applied electrical signal.

Further evidence for a division between energy utilization and energy production in the cochlea comes from deoxyglucose uptake experiments that reveal significant glucose utilization in the same structures containing the Na^+,K^+-ATPase, but considerably less glucose utilization in the organ of Corti (Pujol, Sans, & Calas, 1981; Ryan, Goodwin, Nigel, & Sharp, 1982; Ryan & Sharp, 1982). The division of labor between stria vascularis and the organ of Corti permits the organ of Corti to be avascular. This provides two benefits for hearing. The first is to reduce the mass of the organ of Corti which helps to improve its sensitivity to acoustic stimulation. The second benefit is that the possibility of detecting cardiovascular sounds is reduced.

The force generating mechanism for outer hair cell electromotility is thought to be driven by the receptor potential. The receptor potential results from the modulation of the standing current that occurs when the stereocilia are bent as a result of cochlear partition displacement. The cochlear partition describes the basilar membrane together with the organ of Corti. The electromotile response is thought to provide a positive mechanical feedback that increases the movement of the cochlear partition near threshold (Geisler, 1986; Gold, 1948; Neely & Kim, 1983). The forces associated with this mechanical nonlinearity may be transmitted back to the ear canal in the form of synchronous otoacoustic emissions. High gain, positive feedback systems are inherently unstable and must be kept under control to prevent oscillations. Failure to keep the energy under control could lead to spontaneous otoacoustic emissions. Multiple rows of outer hair cells may help to stabilize the cochlear parti-

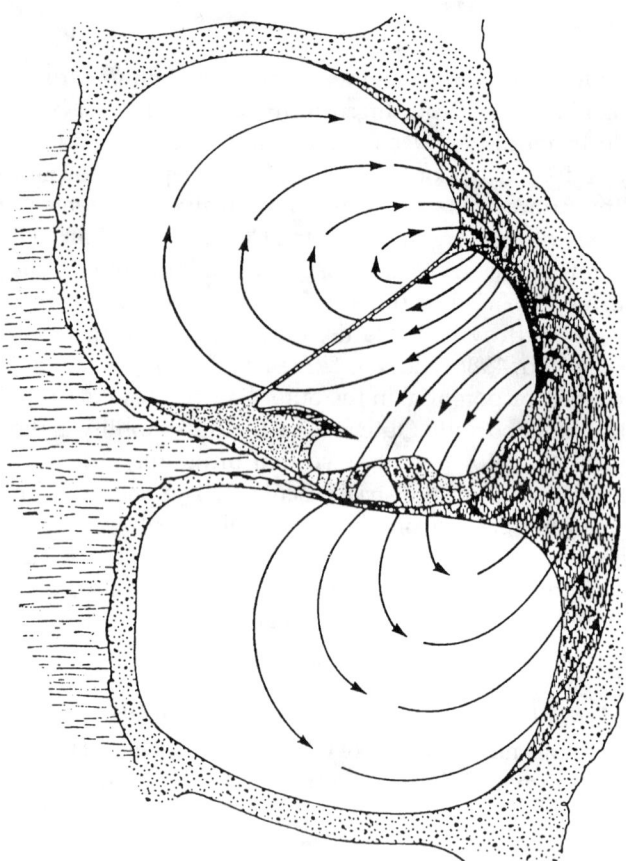

Figure 1–1. Schematic of the electrical environment that powers outer cell electromotility (from Zidanic & Brownell, 1990). The standing (or silent) current is represented in terms of current density field lines. The energy from oxidative phosphorylation in the lateral wall of scala media is used to establish an electrochemical gradient across the organ of Corti. The modulation of the silent current results in outer cell receptor potentials which are thought to drive rapid electromotility in vivo.

tion as random mechanical movements that might trigger oscillations with one row would have to be considerably larger to produce the same result with multiple rows. The three rows typically found in the organ of Corti may represent a balance between increasing the number of rows for stability and the deleterious effect of increasing the mass of the cochlear partition.

Frequency Response

Outer hair cells can move at rates no muscle cell is capable of. They have been monitored following electrical stimulation well into the audio frequency range (Ashmore & Brownell, 1986; Evans, 1988; Evans et al, 1989; Zenner, Zimmerman, & Gitter, 1987). The magnitude of the movements are greatest for low frequencies and decrease with frequency. Some concern has been expressed over the fact that the magnitude of the electrically evoked OHC length changes measured in vitro does not approach the magnitude of threshold cochlear partition movements until the stimulus voltage reaches a value in excess of receptor potentials measured in vivo (Santos-Sacchi, 1989). The same concern calls into question the role of the outer hair cells in the generation of otoacoustic emissions particularly when some stimulated otoacoustic emissions have been measured in response to acoustic stimulation well below the threshold for hearing (Wilson, 1979; Zwicker & Manley, 1981). The movements of isolated outer hair cells are governed by the mechanical properties of the outer hair cell and the electromotile force-generating mechanism (Steele & Jen, 1988). The transfer of force and the resulting movements of the cochlear partition will be determined by its mechanical properties. The mechanical properties of the cochlear partition are different than, and encompass the mechanical properties of, the isolated outer hair cell. It is possible that the outer hair cell undergoes no length change in vivo and that isometric changes in hair cell force are transmitted directly to the cochlear partition. The important feature of the rapid outer hair cell electromotility in isolated cells is that the force generating mechanism can operate at high frequencies.

Asymmetries in Movement

Hyperpolarizing pulses injected into the cell cause the free end (or ends) of the cell to elongate while depolarization results in a shortening (Brownell 1983; Brownell, 1984; Brownell et al, 1985; Santos-Sacchi, 1989; Santos-Sacchi & Dilger, 1988). Extracellular stimulation follows the same basic rules in that the free ends of the cell move in the same direction as the transcellularly applied potential gradient (Brownell, 1984; Brownell et al, 1985; Brownell & Kachar, 1986; Evans, 1990; Evans et al, 1989; Kachar et al, 1986). Transcellularly applied alternating potential gradients have produced symmetric displacements at low frequencies (Brownell & Kachar, 1986; Kachar, Brownell, Altschuler, & Fex, 1986) and nonlinear "DC" responses at high frequencies (Brownell, 1983; Brownell, 1984, Brownell et al, 1985). Recent investigations of response asymmetries (Evans, 1988; Evans, 1990; Evans et al, 1989; Santos-Sacchi, 1989) confirm that the outer hair cell can produce nonlinear asymmetric displacements.

The amount of mechanical rectification seems to be governed by the holding potential (Santos-Sacchi, 1989). There is a range of membrane potentials around which the mechanical response is linear, but when held near −70 mV elongation saturates and shortening dominates. If the membrane potential of transcellularly stimulated cells is considerably less than −70 mV, the mechanical response is likely to be in the linear range. Since the in vivo "resting" potential of outer hair cells appears to be around −70 mV (Dallos et al, 1982; Russell & Sellick, 1983), it is likely that the nonlinear response asymmetries are presented in the living cochlea. Response nonlinearities are necessary in order to account for certain types of evoked otoacoustic emission such as distortion products.

Rapid "DC" displacements of the basilar membrane have been measured (LePage, 1987) in response to tone bursts between 55 and 75 dB SPL. The "DC" displacements may reflect an interaction between the nonlinear nature of outer hair cell electromotility and the inherent rectification present in the receptor potential generator mechanism (Dallos et al, 1982; Russell & Sellick, 1983). Cumulative displacement shifts of the basilar membrane in response to repeated tone bursts have also been measured (LePage, 1987). These may reflect longer time constant mechanical events that could represent an interaction between volume control mechanisms in the outer hair cell and the architectonics of the organ of Corti.

THE ARCHITECTONICS OF THE ORGAN OF CORTI

Outer hair cells are found in the precisely organized cellular matrix of the organ of Corti. The cells in most organs (e.g., liver, heart, skin, retina, maculae, and cristae of the vestibular system) are tightly packed with only 20 to 40 nm separating one cell from the next (Traynelis & Dingledine, 1989). The organ of Corti, in contrast, contains large fluid-filled spaces (see Fig. 1–2). The spaces of Nuel around the outer hair cells provide up to 1000 nm separation between cells and impart the striking colonnade appearance seen in scanning electron micrographs. This organization allows outer hair cell length changes to occur without having to work against the mechanical restrictions imposed by closely packed neighboring cells. Loose attachments with adjacent cells would impede the movement of the lateral cytoplasmic membrane during length changes. The free space can also accommodate diameter changes associated with outer hair cell length changes.

The fluid space around outer hair cells is bordered by the reticular lamina apically and the cell bodies of Deiter's cells basally. The reticular lamina is formed by the apical ends of the hair cells and mechanically

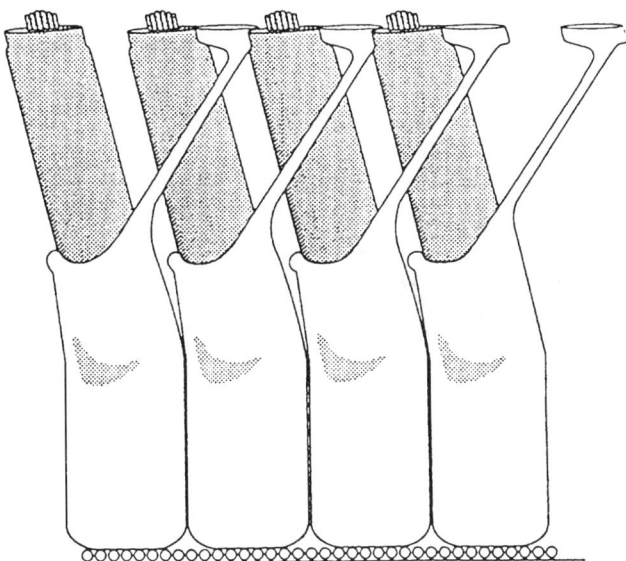

Figure 1–2. Drawing of a portion of a single row of outer hair cells and associated Deiter's cells as viewed from the otic capsule looking toward the modiolus. The apical or high frequency end of the cochlea is to the right, lower frequencies are to the left. The three longitudinal domains of the organ of Corti are from top to bottom: (1) the reticular lamina, (2) the fluid space between the reticular lamina, and (3) the Deiter's cell body layer. The reticular lamina is composed of the apical ends of the hair cells together with the ends of the Deiter's cells phalangeal processes that interdigitate between them. The Deiter's cells sit on the basilar membrane (represented by the row of small circles as its constituent fibers project from the plane of the figure).

rigid extensions of the Deiter's cells that interdigitate between the hair cells (Fig. 1–2). Extremely well developed, tight junctional complexes join the cells where they make contact. The tight junctions contribute toward making the reticular lamina rigid and prevent the mixing of fluids on either side of the reticular lamina. The outer hair cell's apical end is firmly anchored in the reticular lamina while its basal end makes contact with afferent and efferent nerve terminals. The basal end with its attached neural processes rests in a cuplike indentation of a Deiter's cell. The structural integrity of the layer of Deiter's cell bodies is provided by their cytoskeletal elements, the close packing of the cells, and the basilar membrane on which they sit.

The outer hair cells and the thin processes of the Deiter's cells bridge the distance across the fluid space in the organ of Corti. The Deiter's cell process contains a cytoskeletal core that extends from the reticular lamina through the cell body to the basal end of the cell where it rests on basilar membrane. Mechanical probing of the Deiter's cell process reveals that it has little if any compressive strength (WE Brownell, personal observations). Even if it possessed compressive rigidity, the fact that it angles toward the basal end of the cochlear spiral and bends freely about the point of attachment with the Deiter's cell body means that it alone could not prevent the reticular lamina coming closer to the basilar membrane. The separation between the reticular lamina and the Deiter's cell bodies must, therefore, be maintained by outer hair cells. The need for outer hair cells to maintain the separation can be appreciated by imagining the vibrations of the cochlear partition during acoustic stimulation. Since it is crucial that the movements be transmitted to the stereocilia anchored in the reticular lamina, it is understandable as to why the outer hair cells must have sufficient rigidity to withstand the longitudinal compressive forces associated with such movements. The compressive forces of the outer hair cell acting against the tensile properties of the Deiter's cell processes will contribute to the overall compliance of that portion of the cochlear partition.

THE INTRACELLULAR DOMAINS OF THE OUTER HAIR CELL

The shape and static mechanical properties of most animal cells are determined by a network of long chain molecules that are collectively called a cytoskeleton (Alberts et al, 1983). It can be argued on theoretical grounds that the presence of a cytoskeleton would be an impediment to rapid movement. This argument gains support from the fact that there is often an absence or depolymerization of the cytoskeleton in cells or portions of the cell undergoing rapid movements. For instance, immediately before the rapid phase of mitosis the cytoskeleton of the dividing cell depolymerizes and repolymerizes after telophase (Alberts et al, 1983). The very ability of the outer hair cell to change its length requires that it be mechanically flexible. Yet, the structural integrity of the organ of Corti requires that the cell possess considerable compressive rigidity along its major axis. Mammalian hearing imposes on the outer hair cell what seem to be conflicting requirements of mechanical stiffness while at the same time being able to move at acoustic frequencies. By segregating the cytoskeletal structures at the base and the apex of the cell, the outer hair cell leaves the region between the nucleus and the cuticular plate free to move in response to the force generator for the electromotile response.

Ultrastructural and histochemical studies reveal organelles and a structural organization that distinguish the outer hair cell not only from other hair cells but from any other cell so far described. It has a distinctive cylindrical shape with an eccentrically placed nucleus (Fig. 1–3). But it is in the distribution of its cytoskeletal molecules that it displays a dramatic difference with other animal cells. The stereocilia and cuticular plate are

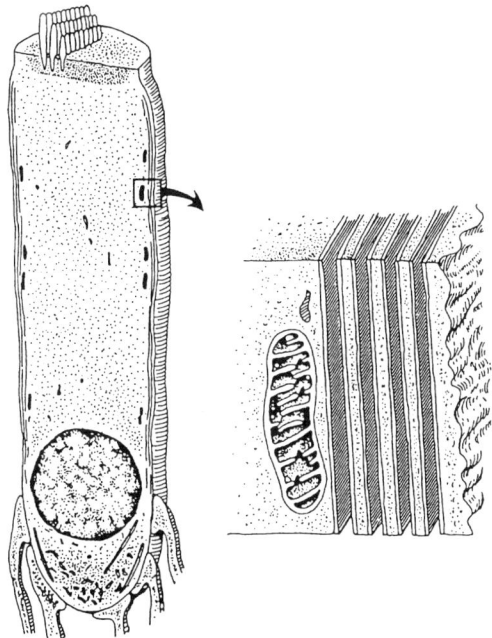

Figure 1–3. Outer hair cell morphology. The general organization of the outer hair cell is shown on the left and a blowup of the cell's cortex is portrayed on the right. The smooth unbroken membranes of the laminated cisternal system are based on the recent description of Evans (1990). Filamentous structures (not portrayed) that may contain actin (Flock, 1988) can be found in the space between the lateral cytoplasmic membrane and the outermost subsurface cistern (see Fig. 1–4). Stereociliar actin filaments are embedded in the cuticular plate at the top of the cell. Cytoskeletal elements are also found in the infranuclear or synaptic region but not in the central cytoplasmic core of the cell between the cuticular plate and the nucleus.

densely packed with actin and other long chain structural molecules. Intermediate filaments and microtubules can be found in the infranuclear region as well. The same studies that demonstrate the presence of structural proteins at the two poles of the cell reveal the axial cytoplasm between the cuticular plate and the nucleus to be remarkably free of cytoskeletal elements (Flock, 1988; Flock, Bretscher, & Weber, 1982; Flock, Flock, & Ulfendahl, 1986; Hackney & Furness, 1989; Slepecky & Chamberlain, 1985; Zenner, 1980). It is the portion of the cell between the nucleus and the cuticular plate that undergoes deformation in response to electrical stimuli. It is unlikely an accident of nature that no significant cytoskeletal organization can be found here.

HYDRAULIC SUPPORT IN THE OUTER HAIR CELL

Nature arrived at a novel solution to the mechanical requirements imposed on the outer hair cell by replacing the cytoskeleton with an hydraulic skeleton. The outer hair cell's subplasma lamina (Bannister, Dodson, Astbury, & Douek, 1988; Lim, Hanamure, & Ohashi, 1989) immediately below the lateral plasma membrane provides a flexible elastic cortex that is stabilized by the positive hydrostatic pressure of the cell's cytoplasm. The formation of a "hydroskeleton" is a structural solution to the problem of how to achieve stiffness with flexible, tensile elements. A hydrostatic supportive system consists of a fluid under pressure in the container wherein the fluid acts as the compression-resisting component and the container alone resists tension. Wainwright (1970) has summarized the functional morphology of hydraulic support systems in animals. The six features that he discusses are easily recognized features of the outer hair cell's morphology (see Fig. 1–4).

1. The outer hair cell has tension and compression resisting elements. The subplasma lamina (Bannister et al, 1988; Flock, 1988; Lim et al, 1989) together with the laminated cisternal system represent the tension resisting elements. The cell's cytoplasm is the compression resisting element.

2. The compression component (the cytoplasm) is the most volumous component in the cell and it extends the length of the cell. The conventional cytoskeletal elements of the outer hair cell are segregated into specific intracellular domains in the base and apex of the cell and do not extend the length of the cell. This contrasts with the cytoskeletal elements that serve as compression units in other cells [e.g., the Deiter's and pillar cells (Hackney & Furness, 1989; Slepecky & Chamberlain, 1983)].

3. A compressive resisting filament free cytoplasm is located at the outer hair cell's central core. An additional structure is found centrally only in the guinea pig outer hair cells and only in cells from the apical region of the cochlea (Carlisle et al, 1989). These cells have actin contain-

ing filaments in their central core that span the distance between the cuticular plate and the nucleus. The organization of these filaments does not favor a compression resisting role.

4. The circumferentially oriented (Bannister et al, 1988; Holly & Ashmore, 1988b; Lim et al, 1989) tension resisting component (Fig. 1–4) extends from the base to the apex in a specialized area of the cell cortex. Additional tension resisting material is found in the cuticular plate-stereociliar complex and infranuclear synaptic region.

5. The tensile material is peripheral.

6. The outer hair cell undergoes 3-dimensional changes in shape. The organization of the subplasma lamina and laminated cisternal system (Bannister et al, 1988; Flock, 1988; Holley & Ashmore, 1988b; Lim et al, 1989) have a crossed-helical arrangement of fibrils that allows for flexibility and strength. There is even evidence for the presence of polysaccharide moieties in the cortical structures of the outer hair cell (Gil-Loyzaga & Brownell, 1988). Animal structures with high tensile strength are made up of high molecular weight protein and polysaccharide moieties whose strongly anisodiametric molecules impart strength along their major axis (Wainwright, 1970).

One consequence of a hydraulic support system based on cylinders is that as the cylinder becomes longer the hydrostatic pressures required to resist longitudinal compressive forces must become larger. This is because of the greater tendency for long structures to shear (bend) while shorter, proportionately wider, structures do not. When the tendency to shear is considered, the effective compressive strength of a cylinder is inversely related to its length. Long, cylindrical, pressure vessels must be stabilized by larger hydrostatic pressures in order to resist the shear that might result from longitudinal compressive forces. Greater hydrostatic pressure in the longer, more apical, outer hair cells may begin to exceed the ability of the "circumferentially" oriented tensile elements in the lateral wall to withstand the longitudinal component of the turgor pressure. Additional tensile elements may be required to withstand the longitudinal stress. The central, actin containing, core described in the longer outer hair cells found closer to the apex of the guinea pig cochlea (Carlisle et al, 1989) may provide the requisite longitudinal tensile strength to resist the increased turgor pressure.

ELECTROMOTILITY AND CELL TURGOR

Cell turgor is required in order that the pressure gradients responsible for the electromotile response can be communicated to the ends of the cell (Brownell & Winston, 1989). Some mechanism must render the outer hair cell's cytoplasm slightly hyperosmotic (Brownell, Imredy, & Shehata, 1989a; Brownell, Shehata, & Imredy, 1989b). This mechanism may be

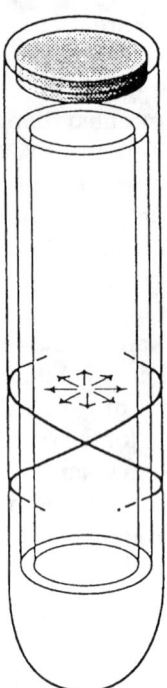

Figure 1–4. Schematic of outer hair cell as a pressure vessel. "Circumferential" tensile elements are indicated by oppositely oriented helices in the lateral walls of the cell (Bannister et al, 1988; Flock, 1988; Holley & Ashmore, 1986; Lim et al, 1989). The radially oriented arrows indicate the cytoplasm's positive hydrostatic pressure. The outer hair cell's turgor pressure is most likely based on a slightly hyperosmotic cytoplasm that "inflates" the cell.

related to the usually high concentration of glycogen in its cytoplasm (Duval & Hukee, 1976; Thalmann, 1975; Thalmann, 1972; Thalmann, Thalmann, & Comegys, 1972). There is a uniform increase in outer hair cell glycogen concentration from the base to the apex of the cochlea. If glycogen contributes to the osmotic pressure of the cytoplasm then outer hair cells near the apex may have a higher turgor pressure.

The outer hair cell can be viewed as a pressure vessel (Fig. 1–4) containing a mechanism for generating pressure gradients at acoustic frequencies. Evidence for the existence of pressure gradients within the axial cytoplasm comes from direct observation of the movement of cellular organelles (Brownell & Kachar, 1986; Holley & Ashmore, 1988a; Kachar, Brownell, Altschuler, & Fex, 1986) in this region. Their movement can only result from pressure gradients particularly in the absence of cytoskeletal elements that might communicate movement directly (Fig. 1–5). The hydrostatic pressure of the outer hair cell makes it a mechanical unit. Changes in the pressure most likely provide the force needed for locomotion. Evidence for the importance of cell turgor for electromotility and otoacoustic emissions comes from manipulations that change hydrostatic the outer hair cell's cytoplasm.

SLOW CHANGES IN OUTER HAIR CELL VOLUME AND TURGOR

Volume Increases

Goldstein and Mizukoshi (1967) were the first to isolate outer hair cells and demonstrate their ability to change shape. They replaced the bathing media,

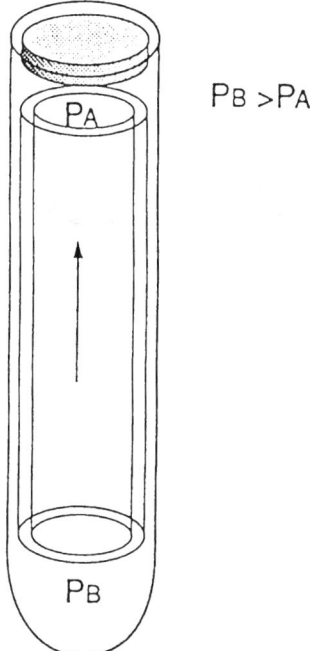

Figure 1–5. Pressure gradients in the axial portion of the cytoplasm are required to explain the movement of cytoplasm associated with rapid electromotility. Pressure effects could be transmitted to the cochlear partition even if the cell is isometrically constrained in situ.

which resembled perilymph, with a high potassium "artificial endolymph" and described the resulting shape change as an increase in cell volume that resembled the increase observed on reducing the osmolarity of the bathing media by dilution with distilled water. Goldstein and Mizukoshi's observations have been confirmed by a number of laboratories which also demonstrated the volume increase to be reversible (Brownell et al, 1989a; Brownell et al, 1989b; Dulon, Aran, & Schacht, 1987; Flock et al, 1986; Ulfendahl, 1988; Ulfendahl & Slepecky, 1988; Zenner, 1986; Zenner, Wolfgang, & Gitter, 1988; Zenner et al, 1985). These chemically induced shape changes follow a time course that is considerably longer than that of rapid electromotility and for this reason they are thought to represent a different type of motile process. Several laboratories have speculated that they result from conventional contractile events triggered by the depolarization of the membrane potential that occurs when the bathing media (with its low potassium concentration) is replaced by the high potassium media. We have examined reversible volume increases stimulated by low ionic strength sugar solutions (Brownell et al, 1989a; Brownell et al, 1989b). The magnitude and time course of the sugar induced shape changes are virtually indistinguishable from those elicited by high extracellular potassium. Morphometric analysis reveals that both the sugar and potassium manipulations lead to increased cell volume with no change in the cell surface area. The low ionic strength sugar solutions hyperpolarize the cells (Brownell et al, 1989b) demonstrating that the slow volume increase need not result from membrane depolarization. The length changes associated with all forms of outer hair cell volume increase is most likely a passive event associated with the solid geometry of cylinders. The only way a cylinder can increase its volume without increasing its surface area is to move toward a spherical shape, so the cylinder becomes shorter and fatter.

The volume increase is most likely the result of an increase in the hydrostatic pressure of the cytoplasm. An increase in the concentration of a solute in the extracellular media leads to an increase in the intracellular concentration of that substance, if the cell's cytoplasmic membrane is permeable to that substance. Unless another substance exits the cell, the cytoplasmic osmolarity will increase and with it the hydrostatic pressure of the cytoplasm. The circumferential tensile strength of the outer hair cell's lateral cortex restores the cell to its elongated shape as the increased hydrostatic pressure that causes the volume increase is reduced on restoring the cell to its normal bathing media. While high potassium environments often lead to volume increases in animal cells with conventional cytoskeletons, osmotically balanced sugar solutions do not. These observations suggest the outer hair cell may possess a unique mechanism for cell volume control that involves permeability changes to nonelectrolytes. The possibility that the outer hair cell membrane can be made permeable to relatively large molecules may explain their nonvesicular uptake of exogenous horseradish peroxidase (Leake-Jones & Snyder, 1987; Siegel & Brownell, 1986).

Volume Decreases

Pharmacological and electrical manipulations can also result in the outer hair cell losing volume. Slow electrically induced changes may be observed with voltage clamp manipulations using tight-seal, whole-cell electrodes. Sustained depolarization leads to a loss of fluid and, once depleted, sustained hyperpolarization leads to an increase of fluid as the cell regains its original shape (Brownell et al, 1989a; Brownell et al, 1989b; Brownell & Winston, 1989). The cells crenulate and flatten as they lose turgor. Rapid movements, evoked by voltage pulses, eventually disappear as the cells lose their turgor during sustained depolarization but return after moving the holding potential to hyperpolarizing values. The dependence of the rapid movements on a normal cytoplasmic pressure is consistent with a mechanism that requires hydraulic transmission of cytoplasmic pressure changes.

Extracellular and intracellular application of salycilates (the active ingredient in aspirin) interferes with the maintenance of outer hair cell turgidity (Brownell et al, 1989a; Brownell et al, 1989b). The cells crenulate and flatten in the same way they do when losing volume with sustained depolarization in voltage clamp. Sustained hyperpolarization is often not able to return the cells to their turgid appearance. This may be associated with the fact that many cells also show an increase in their membrane conductance during aspirin toxicity. Ototoxic doses of aspirin are known to block otoacoustic emissions (Long & Tubis, 1988; McFadden & Plattsmier, 1984). The fact that aspirin blocks both outer hair cell electromotility and otoacoustic emissions is one of the strongest arguments for the role of the outer hair cell in the generation of otoacoustic emissions.

SUMMARY

Analyzing the architectonics of the organ of Corti in light of new knowledge about both the static and dynamic mechanics of the outer hair cell suggest that we should no longer view the outer hair cell as being mechanically supported by Deiter's cells. An integrative view of the structure suggests the compressive strength of the outer hair cell works with the tensile strength of the Deiter's cell process to stabilize and integrate the structure. The outer hair cell supports the Deiter's cell as much as the Deiter's cell supports the outer hair cell. The organ of Corti contains the structural features of the geodesic dome in which short rods with compressive strength are integrated with cables possessing tensile strength. Such structures have "tensegrity" or integrity (Buckminster Fuller, 1975; Roland & Frei, 1965). Structures organized around such interactions are low in mass and can be easily deformed without being damaged.

The measurement of otoacoustic emissions followed by the demonstration of outer hair cell electromotility occurred at a pivotal moment for the evolution of our understanding of the inner ear. The ability of a source of acoustic energy in the organ of Corti to explain a variety of experimental observations on cochlear mechanics, including the generation of otoacoustic emissions, helped to establish a role for bidirectional transduction in the cochlea and permitted the hearing science community to embrace the motor capabilities of the inner ear.

Acknowledgments: Work supported by Office of Naval Research, task 441k704.

REFERENCES

Alberts B, Bray D, Lewis J, Raff M, Roberts K, and Watson JD. Molecular Biology of the Cell. New York: Garland, 1983.

Ashmore JF and Brownell WE. Kilohertz movements induced by electrical stimulation in outer hair cells isolated from the guinea pig cochlea. J Physiol 1986;377:41 P.

Ashmore JF and Meech RW. Ionic basis of membrane potential in outer hair cells of guinea pig cochlea. Nature 1986;322:368–371.

Assad JA, Hacohen N, and Corey DP. Voltage dependence of adaptation and active bundle movement in bullfrog saccular hair cells. Proc Natl Acad Sci USA 1989;86:2918–2922.

Bannister LH, Dodson HC, Astbury AF, and Douek EE. The cortical lattice: a highly ordered system of subsurface filaments in guinea pig cochlear outer hair cells. Prog Brain Res 1988;74:213–219.

Békésy G. Experiments in Hearing. New York: McGraw-Hill, 1960.

Brown MC and Nuttal AL. Efferent control of cochlear inner hair cell responses in the guinea pig. J Physiol 1984,354:625–646.

Brown MC, Nuttall AL, and Masta RI. Intracellular recordings from cochlear inner hair cells: effects of stimulation of the crossed olivocochlear efferents. Science 1983;222:69–72.

Brownell WE. Cochlear transduction: An integrative model and review. Hear Res 1982;6:335–360.

Brownell WE. Observations on a motile response in isolated outer hair cells. In Webster WR and Aitken LM, Eds. Mechanisms of Hearing. Monash University Press, 1983:5–10.

Brownell WE. Microscopic observation of cochlear hair cell motility. Scanning Electron Microsc 1984/III:1401–1406.

Brownell WE. Outer hair cell motility and cochlear frequency selectivity. In Moore BCJ and Patterson RD, Eds. Auditory Frequency Selectivity. New York: Plenum Press, 1986:109–120.

Brownell WE, Bader CR, Bertrand D, and de Ribaupierre Y. Evoked mechanical responses of isolated cochlear outer hair cells. Science 1985;227:194–196.

Brownell WE, Imredy JP, and Shehata W. Stimulated volume changes in mammalian outer hair cells. Proc Ann Int Conf IEEE-Eng Med Biol Soc 1989a;11: 1344–1345.

Brownell WE, Kachar B. Outer hair cell motility: A possible electro-kinetic mechanism. In Allen JB, Hall JL, Hubbard AE, Neely ST, and Tubis A, Eds. Peripheral Auditory Mechanisms. New York: Springer-Verlag, 1986:369–376.

Brownell WE, Manis PB, Zidanic M, and Spirou GA. Acoustically evoked radial current densities in scala tympani. J Acoust Soc Am 1983;74:792–800.

Brownell WE, Shehata W, and Imredy JP. Slow electrically and chemically evoked volume changes in guinea pig outer hair cells. In Akkas N, Ed. Biomechanics of Active Movement and Deformation of Cells. New York: Springer-Verlag, 1989b:493–498.

Brownell WE and Winston JB. Slow electrically evoked volume changes in guinea pig outer hair cells. Abstracts of the Midwinter Research Meeting of the Association for Research in Otolaryngology. 1989;12:138–139.

Brownell WE, Zidanic M, and Spirou GA. Standing currents and their modulation in the cochlea. In Altschuler R, Hoffman D, and Bobbin R, Eds. Neurobiology of Hearing: The Cochlea. New York: Raven Press, 1986:91–107.

Carlisle L, Thorne PR, Zajic G, Altschuler RA, and Schacht J. A comparative study of actin filaments in cochlear hair cells: outer hair cells in the apex of the guinea pig cochlea contain a unique ultrastructural feature. In Wilson JP and Kemp DT, Eds. Cochlear Mechanisms Structure, Function and Models. New York: Plenum Press, 1989:21–28.

Crawford AC and Fettiplace R. The mechanical properties of ciliary bundles of turtle cochlear hair cells. J Physiol (Lond) 1985;364:359–379.

Dallos P, Santos-Sacchi J, and Flock A. Intracellular recordings from cochlear outer hair cells. Science 1982;218:582–584.

Drescher DG and Kerr TP. Na^+,K^+-activated adenosine triphosphatase and carbonic anhydrase: Inner ear enzymes of ion transport. In Dresher DG, Ed. Auditory Biochemistry. Springfield: Charles C Thomas, 1985;436–472.

Dulguerov P, Zidanic M, and Brownell WE. Potassium gradients in scala tympani of the guinea pig in the absence of sound stimulation. Soc. Neurosci. Abst. 1985;15:245.

Dulon D, Aran J-M, and Schacht J. Osmotically induced motility of outer hair cells: implications for Meniere's disease. Arch Otorhinolaryngol 1987;244: 104–107.

Duval AJ III and Hukee MJ. Delineation of cochlear glycogen by electron microscopy. Ann Otol Rhinol Laryngol 1976;85:234–246.

Evans BN. Asymmetries in outer hair cell electro-mechanical responses. Abstracts of the Midwinter Meeting of the Association for Research in Otolaryngology, 1988;11:29.

Evans BN. (in press). *In vitro* correlates of outer hair cell vulnerability: Electromechanical and ultrastructural observations. Hear Res 1990.

Evans B, Dallos P, and Hallworth R. Asymmetries in motile responses of outer hair cells in simulated *in vivo* conditions. In Wilson JP and Kemp DT, Eds. Cochlear Mechanisms Structure Function and Models. New York: Plenum Press, 1989:205–206.

Flock Å. Do sensory cells in the ear have a motile function? Prog Brain Res 1988;74:297–304.

Flock Å, Bretscher A, and Weber K. Immunohistochemical localization of several cytoskeletal proteins in inner ear sensory and supporting cells. Hear Res 1982,6:75–89.

Flock Å, Flock B, and Ulfendahl M. Mechanisms of movement in outer hair cells and a possible structural basis. Arch Otorhinolaryngol 1986;243:83–90.

Fuller, B. R. Synergetics. New York: MacMillan, 1975.

Geisler CD. A model of the effect of outer hair cell motility on cochlear vibrations Hear Res 1986,24:125–132.

Gil-Loyzaga PE and Brownell WE. Wheat germ agglutinin and *Helix Pomatia* agglutinin lectin binding on cochlear hair cells. Hear Res 1988;34:149–156.

Gitter AH, Zenner HP, and Fromter E. Membrane potential and ion channels in isolated outer hair cells of guinea pig cochlea. ORL 1986; 48:68–75.

Gold T. The physical basis of the action of the cochlea. Proc R Soc Lond B Biol Sci 1948;135:492–498.

Goldstein AJ and Mizukoshi O. Separation of the organ of Corti into its component cells. Ann Otol Rhinol Laryngol 1967;76:414–426.

Hackney CM and Furness DN. Observations on the cytoskeleton and related structures of mammalian cochlear hair cells. In Wilson JP and Kemp DT, Eds. Cochlear Mechanisms Structure, Function and Models. New York: Plenum Press 1989:11–20.

Holley MD and Ashmore JF. On the mechanism of a high-frequency force generator in outer hair cells isolated from the guinea pig cochlea. Proc R Soc Lond B Biol Sci 1988a;232:413–429.

Holley MD and Ashmore JF. A cytoskeletal spring in cochlear outer hair cells. Nature 1988b,335:635–637.

Jen DH and Steele CR. Electrokinetic model of cochlear hair cell motility. J Acoust Soc Am 1987;82:1667–1678.

Johnstone BM, Patuzzi RB, Syka J, and Sykova E. Stimulus-related potassium changes in the organ of Corti of guinea-pig. J Physiol (Lond) 1989;408:77–92

Kachar B, Brownell WE, Altschuler RA, and Fex J. Electro-kinetic shape changes of cochlear outer hair cells. Nature 1986;322:365–368.

Kemp DT. Stimulated acoustic emissions from within the human auditory system. J Acoust Soc Am 1978;64:1386–1391.

Kerr TP, Ross MD, and Ernst SA. Cellular localization of Na^+,K^+-ATPase in the mammalian cochlear duct: Significance for cochlear fluid balance. Am J Otolaryngol 1982;3:332–338.

Khanna SM and Leonard DGB. Basilar membrane tuning in the cat cochlea. Science 1982;215:305–306.

Kiang NYS, Watanabe T, Thomas EC, and Clark LF. Discharge Patterns of Single Fibers in the Cat's Auditory Nerve. Cambridge; MIT Press, 1965.

Klinke R and Smolder J. Hearing mechanisms in caiman and pigeon. In Bolis L, Keynes R, and Maddrell S, Eds. Comparative Physiology of Sensory Systems. Cambridge University Press, 1984.

Leake-Jones P and Snyder R. Uptake of horseradish peroxidase from perilymph by cochlear hair cells. Hear Res 1987;25:153–171.

LePage EL. Frequency-dependent self-induced bias of the basilar membrane and its potential for controlling sensitivity and tuning in the mammalian cochlea. J Acoust Soc Am 1987;82:139–154.

Lim DJ, Hanamure Y, and Ohashi Y. Structural organization of the mammalian auditory hair cells in relation to micromechanics. In Wilson JP, and Kemp DT, Eds. Cochlear Mechanisms Structure, Function and Models. New York: Plenum Press, 1989:3–10.

Long GR and Tubis A. Modification of spontaneous and evoked otoacoustic emissions and associated psychoacoustic microstructure by aspirin consumption. J Acoust Soc Am 1988;84:1343–1353.

Manley GA, Schulze M, and Oeckinghaus H. Otoacoustic emissions in a song bird. Hear Res 1987;26:257–266.

McFadden D and Plattsmier HS. Aspirin abolishes spontaneous oto-acoustic emissions. J Acoust Soc Am 1984,76:443–448.

Mountain DC. Changes in endolymphatic potential and crossed olivocochlear bundle stimulation alter cochlear mechanics. Science 1980;210:71–72.

Mountain DC. Active filtering by hair cells. In Allen JB, Hall JL, Hubbard AE, Neely ST, and Tubis A, Eds. Peripheral Auditory Mechanisms. New York: Springer-Verlag, 1986.

Neely ST and Kim DO. An active cochlear model showing sharp tuning and high sensitivity. Hear Res 1983;9:123–130.

Palmer AR and Wilson JP. Spontaneous and evoked acoustic emissions in the frog *Rana esculenta*. J Physiol 1981;324:66P.

Pujol R, Sans A, and Calas A. High resolution radioautographic study of the inner ear following *in vivo* tritiated deoxyglucose administration. Eur Neurol 1981;20:157–161.

Rhode WS, Observations on the vibration of the basilar membrane in squirrel monkeys using the Mössbauer technique. J Acoust Soc Am 1971;49:1218–1231.

Rhode WS. Some observations on cochlear mechanics. J Acoust Soc Am 1978;64:158–176.

Robles L, Ruggero MA, and Rich NC. Basilar membrane mechanics at the base of the chinchilla cochlea. I. Input-output functions, tuning curves, and phase responses. J Acoust Soc Am 1986;80:1364–1374.

Roland C. Frei Otto: Tension Structures. New York: Praeger, 1965.

Russell IJ and Sellick PM. Intracellular studies of hair cells in the mammalian cochlea. J Physiol 1978;284:261–290.

Russell IJ and Sellick PM. Low frequency characteristics of intracellularly recorded receptor potentials in mammalian hair cells. J Physiol 1983;338:179–206.

Ryan AF, Goodwin P, Nigel KW, and Sharp F. Auditory stimulation alters the pattern of 2-deoxyglucose uptake in the inner ear. Brain Res 1982;234:213–225.

Ryan AF and Sharp FR. Localization of (^{3}H)2-deoxyglucose at the cellular level using freeze-dried tissue and dry-looped emulsion. Brain Res 1982;252: 177–180.

Santos-Sacchi J. Asymmetry in voltage-dependent movements of isolated outer hair cells from the organ of Corti. J Neurosci 1989;9:2954–2962.

Santos-Sacchi J and Dilger JP. Whole cell currents and mechanical responses of isolated outer hair cells.Hear Res 1988;35:143–150.

Schulte BA and Adams JC. Distribution of immunoreactive Na$^+$, K$^+$-ATPase in gerbil cochlea. J Histochem Cytochem 1989;37:127–134.

Sellick PM, Patuzzi R, and Johnstone BM. Measurement of basilar membrane motion in the guinea pig using the Mossbauer technique. J Acoust Soc Am 1982;72:131–141

Siegel JH and Brownell WE. Synaptic and Golgi membrane recycling in cochlear hair cells. J Neurocytol 1986;15:311–32 8.

Siegel JH and Kim DO. Efferent neural control of cochlear mechanics? Olivocochlear bundle stimulation affects cochlear biomechanical nonlinearity. Hear Res 1982;6:171–182.

Slepecky N and Chamberlain SC. Distribution and polarity of actin in inner ear supporting cells. Hear Res 1983;10:359–370.

Slepecky N and Chamberlain SC. Immuno-electron-microscopic and immunofluorescent localization of cytoskeletal and muscle-like contractile proteins in inner ear sensory cells. Hear Res 1985;20:245–260.

Steele CR and Jen DH. Mechanical analysis of hair cell microstructure and motility. In Wilson JP and Kemp DT, Eds. Cochlear Mechanisms Structure Function and Models. New York: Plenum Press, 1988:67–74.

Strack G, Klinke R, and Wilson JP. Evoked cochlear response in *Caiman crocodilus*. Pfluegers Arch 1981: (Suppl 391):R43.

Thalmann R. Biochemical studies of the auditory system. In Tower DB, Ed. Human Communication and Its Disorders, Vol 3. Raven Press: New York, 1975:31–44.

Thalmann R. Recent refinements of quantitative microchemical analysis of tissues and cells of the inner ear. Acta Otolaryngol 1972:73:160–174.

Thalmann R, Thalmann I, and Comegys TH. Quantitative cytochemistry of the organ of Corti. Dissection, weight determination and analysis of single outer hair cell. Laryngoscope 1972;11:2059–2078.

Traynelis ST and Dingledine R. Role of extracellular space in hyperosmotic suppression of potassium-induced electrographic seizures. J Neurophysiol 1989:61:927–938.

Ulfendahl M. Volume and length changes in outer hair cells of the guinea pig after potassium-induced shortening. Arch Otorhinolaryngol 1988;245: 237–243.

Ulfendahl M and Slepecky N. Ultrastructural correlates of inner ear sensory cell shortening. J Submicrosc Cytol Pathol 1988;20:47–51.

Wainwright SA. Design in hydraulic organisms. Die Naturwissenschaften 1970;57:321–326.
Whitehead ML, Wilson JP, and Baker RJ. The effects of temperature on otoacoustic emission tuning properties. In Moore BCJ and Patterson RD, Eds. Auditory Frequency Selectivity. New York: Plenum Press, 1986:39–48.
Wilson JP. Subthreshold mechanical activity within the cochlea. J Physiol 1979;298:32–33P.
Wit HP, van Dijk P, and Segenhaut JM. An electrical correlate of spontaneous otoacoustic emission in a frog, a preliminary report. In Wilson JP and Kemp DT, Eds. Cochlear Mechanisms Structure, Function and Models. New York: Plenum Press, 1988:341–347.
Zenner HP. Cytoskeletal and muscle like elements in cochlear hair cells. Arch Otorhinolaryngol 1980:230:81–92.
Zenner HP. Motile responses in outer hair cells. Hear Res 1986:22:83–90.
Zenner HP, Wolfgang A, and Gitter AH. Outer hair cells as fast and slow cochlear amplifiers with a bidirectional transduction cycle. Acta Otolaryngol 1988; 105:457–462.
Zenner, HP, Zimmerman U, and Gitter AH. Fast motility of isolated mammalian auditory sensory cells. Biochem Biophys Res Commun 1987:149:304–308.
Zenner HP, Zimmerman U, and Schmitt U. Reversible contraction of isolated mammalian cochlear hair cells. Hear Res 1985;18:127–133.
Zidanic M and Brownell WE. (in press). Low-frequency modulation of the intracochlear potential field: An energy source for the cochlear amplifier. II Valsalva (1990).
Zidanic M and Brownell WE. (in press). The fine structure of the intracochlear potential field. I. The silent current. Biophys J 1990.
Zwicker E and Manley GA. Acoustical responses and suppression-period patterns in guinea pigs. Hear Res 1981;4:43–52.

Acknowledgments: The editorial review of Drs. D. K. Ryugo, W. E. Shehata, E. D. Young, and M. Zidanic is greatly appreciated.

Address reprint requests to: William E. Brownell, Department of Otorhinolaryngology, Louisiana State University School of Medicine, 2020 Gravier Street, Suite A, New Orleans, LA 70112-2234.

2

Chemical Receptors on Outer Hair Cells and Their Molecular Mechanisms

Richard P. Bobbin, Ph.D.
Kresge Hearing Research Laboratory of the South,
Department of Otorhinolaryngology and Biocommunication,
Louisiana State University Medical Center
New Orleans, Louisiana

INTRODUCTION

We know that normal hearing depends on the proper functioning of active and passive cochlear mechanics and that the outer hair cells (OHCs) play a central role in the active mechanics. Various investigations have shown that the efferent nerves that innervate the OHCs influence cochlear mechanics by way of neurotransmitter chemicals released onto the OHCs. In addition, other cells in the organ of Corti and even the OHCs themselves may also release chemicals that act on the OHCs, that is, the chemicals act in a paracrine or autocrine manner. This chapter reviews the mechanisms of action of a few endogenous chemicals that act on OHCs with emphasis on the unique pharmacology of the efferent neurotransmitter, acetylcholine. The eventual goal of such studies is to understand the action of these molecules at the cellular and subcellular level and so understand the molecular mechanisms of cochlear mechanics.

Active and Passive Mechanics

The function of the cochlea is now thought of in terms of an active and passive mechanism as shown schematically in Figure 2–1. The passive mechanism is utilized during sound exposure over 40–60 dB SPL, where sound energy is powerful enough to move the cochlear partition directly.

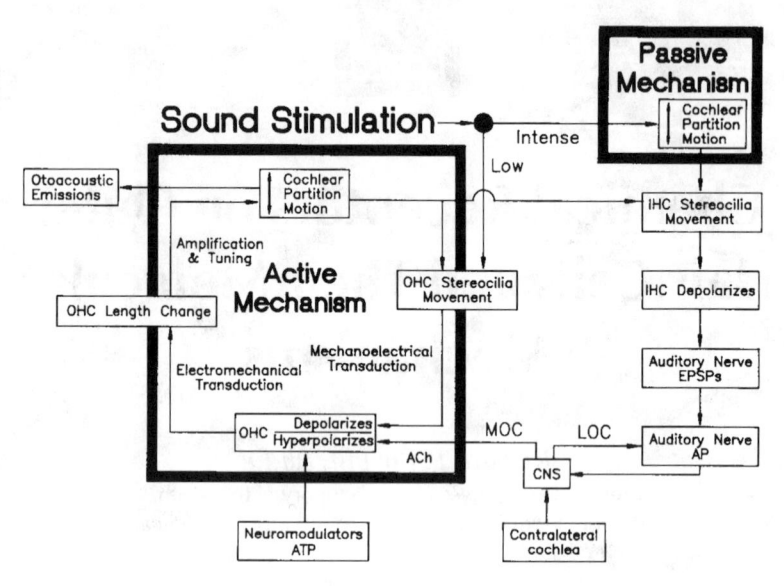

Figure 2–1. Schematic of the action of the passive and active mechanism for cochlear partition mechanics. IHC: inner hair cell; OHC: outer hair cell; LOC: lateral olivocochlear nerve tract; MOC: medial olivocochlear nerve tract; EPSPs: excitatory postsynaptic potentials; AP: action potential; ATP: adenosine triphosphate; ACh: acetylcholine; CNS: central nervous system. (Adapted from Pujol, 1990.)

This results in the movement of inner hair cell (IHC) stereocilia and opening of transduction channels which results in depolarization (less negative or more positive voltage) of the IHCs. Depolarization of the IHCs releases the neurotransmitter (i.e., glutamate) onto the auditory nerve endings which produces action potentials in the auditory nerve fibers. The active mechanism is utilized during low levels of sound exposure (<40 dB SPL) when the sound energy is insufficient to move the cochlear partition directly. Instead, in some unknown fashion, sound at this low level induces movement of the stereocilia on the OHCs. The movement of the OHC stereocilia opens transduction channels and depolarizes the OHCs (i.e., mechanoelectrical transduction). Depolarization of the OHCs changes the length of the OHCs (i.e., electromechanical transduction). This length change then results in amplification by inducing additional movement of the OHC stereocilia and greater depolarization and even greater length change of the OHC. The change in length of the OHC will move the cochlear partition and the greater the OHC length change, the greater the cochlear partition motion. When the movement of the partition is sufficient to induce IHC stereocilia movement, then events as described previously for the passive mechanism will take place, producing action potentials in the auditory nerve. The amplification of the cochlear partition movement by the active mechanism contributes to the energy being transmitted back out through the ossicles in the form of otoacoustic emissions.

The OHCs are the key elements in the active process, with possibly some role for other cells such as Deiters cells (Dulon, 1994, Dulon, Blanchet, & Laffon, 1994; Dulon, Moataz, & Mollard, 1993; Moataz, Saito, & Dulon, 1992). Therefore, the OHC is a good anatomical point for the ear to control its response to sound. This is accomplished through several chemicals that act on the OHCs to alter their ability to change length in response to sound. As the motor of the OHCs is voltage controlled (Santos-Sacchi & Dilger, 1988), the degree of polarization of the OHCs determines the length of the OHCs: the more positive and farther away from its resting potential (@ –60 mV) the greater the shortening. Some chemicals depolarize the OHCs (i.e., membrane potential more positive) and this allows the OHC to shorten to a greater degree in response to sound. Others hyperpolarize the OHCs (i.e., membrane potential more negative) and this makes the OHC shorten less to sound. Other chemicals that affect intracellular chemical messengers are called second messengers (e.g., Ca^{2+}). Second messengers increase or decrease the length change in response to sound through a molecular mechanism inside the cell. The most studied chemicals are those released onto the OHCs from the efferent nerve fibers.

Efferent Innervation

Others have described the innervation of the cochlea by the olivocochlear efferent nerve fibers (e.g., Warr & Guinan, 1979). As shown in Figure 2–2, the medial portion of the olivocochlear efferents (MOC) synapse with the

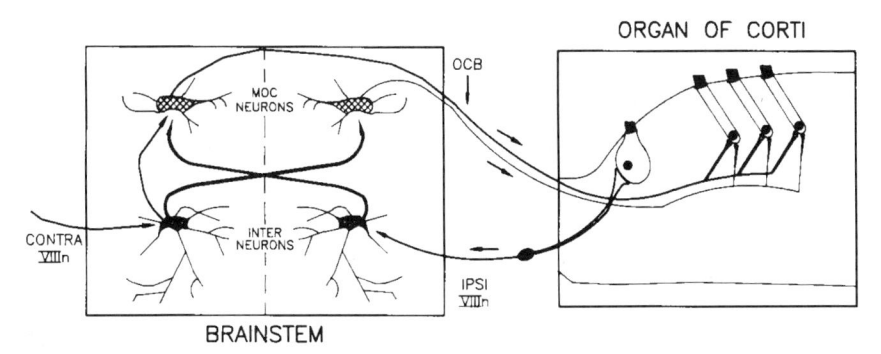

Figure 2–2. Innervation of the organ of Corti and the hair cells by the medial portion (MOC) of the olivocochlear nerve bundle (OCB) which originates in the brain stem. (Adapted from Liberman and T. Kawase, 1992.)

OHCs. Both contralateral and ipsilateral sound activate these MOC efferents and affect the activity of the OHCs by means of released chemical messengers. Thus, MOC nerve fibers play an important role in adjusting the active process. There are thought to be several chemicals involved in the mechanism of action of these efferent nerve fibers (see review by Eybalin, 1993). Here we will discuss only a few of the chemicals, with emphasis on acetylcholine (ACh).

NEUROTRANSMITTERS

Acetylcholine

Antagonists—in Vivo

There is no doubt that acetylcholine (ACh) functions as the primary neurotransmitter that the MOC neurons release onto the OHCs. This evidence comes from the pioneering studies by Guth, Norris, and others (see reviews by Bledsoe, Bobbin, & Puel, 1988; Daigneault, 1981; Eybalin, 1993; Guth, Norris, & Bobbin, 1976). ACh is a neurotransmitter at many locations, for example, the heart, neuromuscular junction. However, it appears that the receptor protein on the OHCs, to which ACh couples, is unique.

The uniqueness of the pharmacology of this ACh receptor protein was suggested in the earliest studies utilizing electrical stimulation of the MOC fibers in the brain stem and applying antagonists of various receptors intracochlearly to the perilymph compartment. Desmedt and Monaco (1960) were the first to demonstrate that strychnine applied to the round window (i.e., into perilymph) blocked the electrically induced action of these efferents (Figure 2–3). They suggested that the receptor protein was similar to the glycine receptor, since at that time strychnine was thought to be a specific blocker of neurotransmitter glycine. However, Churchill, Schuknecht, and Doran (1956) and Schuknecht, Churchill, and Doran (1959) had demonstrated that the efferent fibers stained for cholinesterase, suggesting that the efferent transmitter was ACh. Fex (1968) then demonstrated that curare, an antagonist of the ACh receptor at the neuromuscular junction, applied to the perilymph, blocked the efferents. This was some of the first evidence presented to show that the receptor protein on the OHCs was similar to the ACh receptor protein at the neuromuscular junction (Figure 2–4; because nicotine activates the ACh receptor at the neuromuscular junction, the receptor is called a nicotinic receptor—abbreviated Nm).

Table 2–1 is a partial summary of the pharmacology of this synapse obtained utilizing intracochlear perilymph application of the drugs and

CHEMICAL RECEPTORS ON OUTER HAIR CELLS

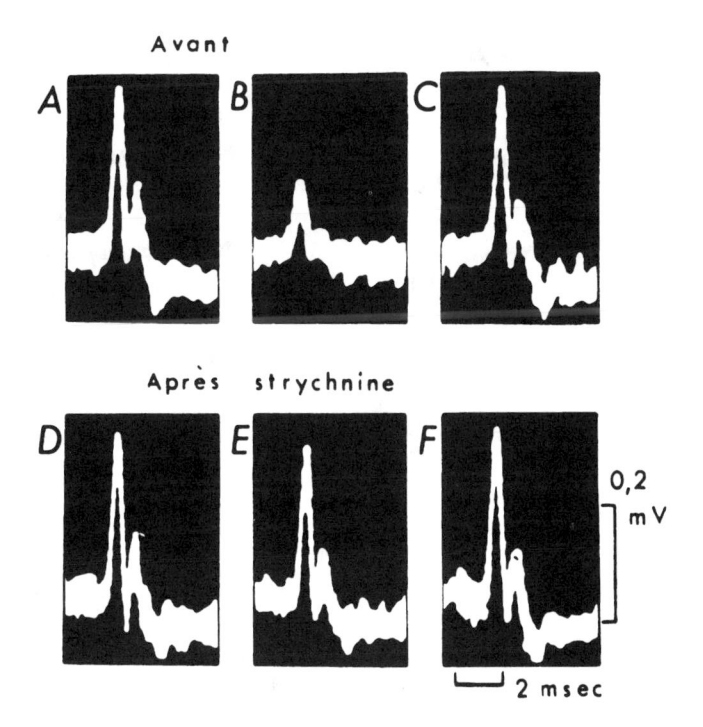

Figure 2–3. Oscilloscope traces showing the responses of the acoustic nerve (round window) stimulated by a click of 20 dB above threshold. Four successive traces are superimposed on each graph in order to show the stability of the response. In **B** and **E**, a train of 30 shocks (30 microseconds, 6 volts) at 300/sec was applied to the bundle of Rasmussen at the level of its decussation 20 msec before the tested click. The olivocochlear inhibition of the click response appears clearly when you compare the traces **B** and **E** to the responses of a single click (not preceded by the train) obtained before (**A** and **D**) and after (**C** and **F**) the stimulation of the bundle of Rasmussen. The administration of strychnine considerably reduced the olivocochlear centrifugal inhibition, but does not affect the response to the single click. (From Desmedt and Monaco, 1960, with permission.) (Translated by author)

electrical stimulation of the MOC efferents in the brain stem (from Bobbin & Konishi, 1971a, 1971b, 1974; Fex & Adams, 1978; & Galley, Klinke, Oertel, Pause, & Storch, 1973). For instance, Konishi and I found that the effects of the efferents could be blocked by atropine, a muscarinic receptor antagonist (the receptor found at the autonomic innervation of glands and smooth muscle and called a muscarinic type of receptor as it is activated by the drug muscarine, abbreviated M). Atropine exhibited less potency than either strychnine or curare. At the time, this unusual block by atropine was tempered by the fact that the quaternary atropine was

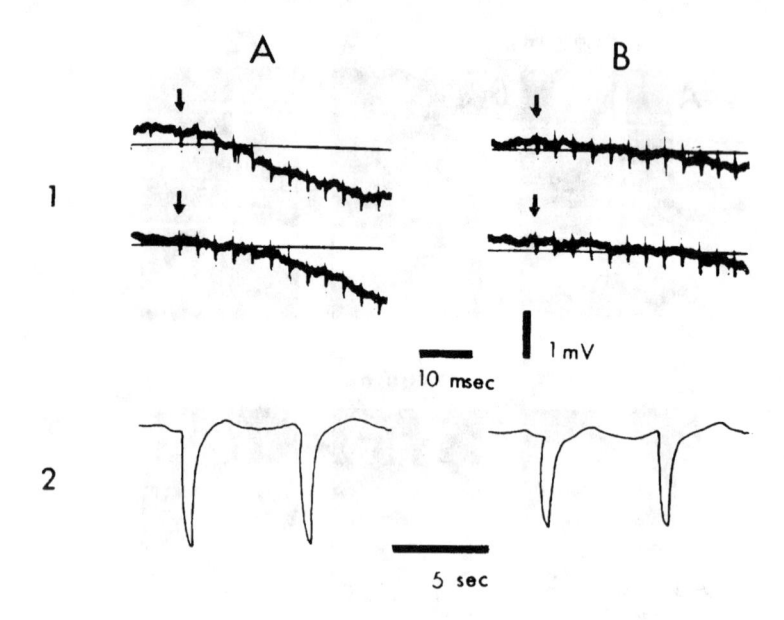

Figure 2–4. Records illustrating the action of d-tubocurarine on centrifugally evoked intracochlear potentials. Row 1 shows the initial time-course of potentials that were evoked by repetitive electrical stimulation of crossed olivo-cochlear fibres. Row 2 shows the full time-course of the potentials of Row 1. All the records were taken with the microelectrode in one position in the scala media. The start of stimulation is indicated by an arrow in Row 1. **A.** Control, artificial perilymph in the scala tympani. **B.** 12.5 minutes later than **A**. Artificial perilymph containing 1.0 μmole (0.7 × 10^{-6} g/ml) d-tubocurarine had, 5–8.5 minutes later than **A**, partly replaced the solution without d-tubocurarine. Note that after the application of d-tubocurarine, the time of rise and the latency of the potentials were prolonged and the amplitude decreased.

Note that voltage calibration is common to all the records, while time calibration is different for the two rows. The ink-writer that produced the records of Row 2 had a rise time constant of 0.15 seconds; d.c. recordings were used for all records. Negativity is downward. (From Fex, 1968, with permission.)

more potent than the tertiary atropine, a finding in harmony with a nicotinic type of receptor. In addition, we found decamethonium more potent than hexamethonium, suggesting that the receptor was like the acetylcholine receptor at the neuromuscular junction (nicotinic receptor, Nm) and less like the acetylcholine receptor at autonomic ganglia (nicotinic, Nn). Others reported that alpha-bungarotoxin, an antagonist at the Nm

TABLE 2–1. A summary listing of antagonists of the effects of electrical stimulation of the MOC on cochlear potentials. Also given is a list of the receptor types and the locations where these antagonists are most selective.

Receptor type	Location	Antagonist of MOC
Nicotinic (Nm)	skeletal muscle	curare, α-BTX, quaternary atropine, decamethonium
Nicotinic (Nn)	autonomic ganglia	hexamethonium
Muscarinic (M)	smooth muscles, glands	atropine
Glycinergic (gly)	central nervous system	strychnine

receptor, also blocked the efferents (Fex & Adams, 1978). Overall, it appeared that the receptor protein on the OHCs was similar to the Nm receptor, yet it was different because it was blocked by so many drugs that acted at other receptors. But because the experimental preparations were so complex, one was not sure where the drugs were acting. For instance, the action of strychnine was attributed to the drug blocking the release of ACh and not due to blocking the receptor (Fex, 1968, p. 183).

An additional problem with studying this efferent/OHC synapse using electrical stimulation of the MOC nerves was the difficult surgery and the instability of the preparation during the experiment. The discovery by Puel and Rebillard (1990) of a method of activating the efferents by sound to the contralateral ear yielded a technique that made the study of the pharmacology much easier. They monitored the effect of the efferents on the distortion product emissions (DPOAEs) which reflect the activity of the OHCs, and demonstrated that DPOAEs were suppressed by contralateral sound (Figure 2–5).

Kujawa, Glattke, Fallon, and Bobbin (1993) duplicated the Puel and Rebillard study and found that the response to contralateral noise was blocked by intracochlearly applied strychnine, curare, and atropine, with atropine being the least potent (Figure 2–6). In addition, the preparation was sufficiently stable so that Kujawa, Glattke, Fallon, & Bobbin (1994a) could generate cumulative dose response curves for the various types of pharmacological agents (Figure 2–7). Utilizing this technique, Kujawa et al. (1994a) demonstrated that the ACh receptor on the OHCs did indeed

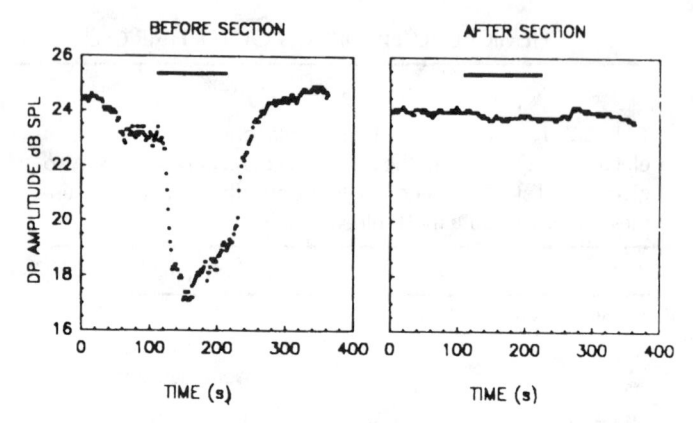

Figure 2-5. Effect of a midline sagittal section of the brainstem on 2F1–F2 DPs recorded at 5 kHz. The **left panel** represents the 2F1–F2 DPs reduction induced by a 100 dB SPL contralateral white noise. The **right panel** shows that after a complete midline sagittal section of the brainstem, the suppressive effect of the contralateral white noise is no longer active. The horizontal bars represent the time during which the contralateral white noise was presented. (From Puel and Rebillard, 1990, with permission.)

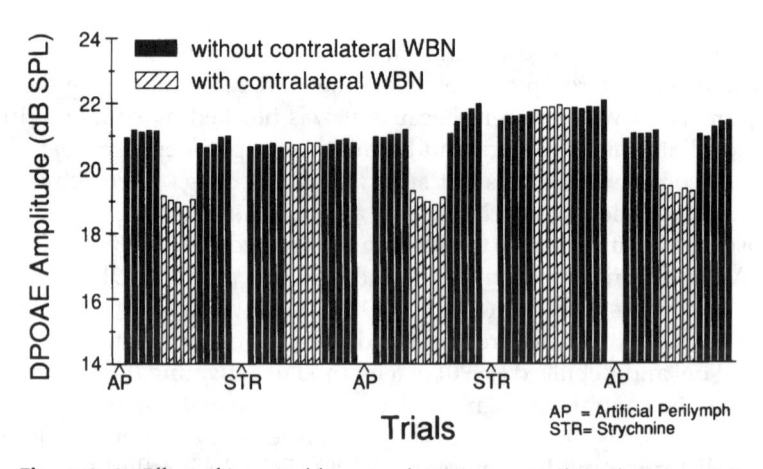

Figure 2-6. Effect of intracochlear strychnine on contralateral suppression of DPOAEs in one representative animal. DPOAE amplitudes are shown after the second control perfusion (artificial perilymph; AP) and after perfusions of 10 μM strychnine (STR) which were followed by artificial perilymph (AP) perfusions that washed out the drug. Each perfusion was 10 minutes in duration; post-perfusion measures are separated by an approximately 25 minute interval during which time the perfusion was completed, post-perfusion measures were taken, and the perfusion pipette was prepared for the next perfusion. Each "trial" represents a 50 spectra average and required 20 seconds to complete. Each set of post-perfusion measures thus required a total of approximately 300 seconds. Graph represents a total time of approximately 2.5 hours. (From Kujawa et al., 1993, with permission.)

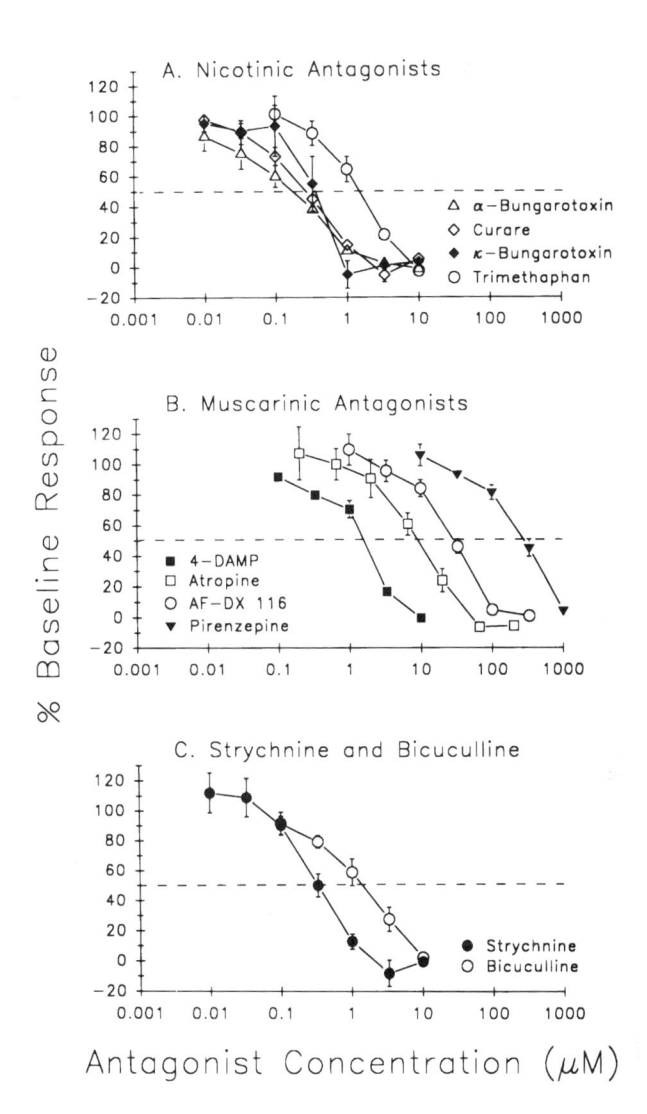

Figure 2-7. Inhibition curves (means ± S.E.) for antagonist blockade of baseline contralateral suppression. Curves associated with nicotinic antagonists are displayed in **panel A**, those associated with the muscarinic antagonists in **panel B** and the curves associated with the nontraditional cholinergic antagonists strychnine and bicuculline are shown in **panel C**. Magnitude of contralateral suppression following the second control perfusion established the baseline response for each animal. Magnitude of suppression as recorded following each concentration of experimental drug was then expressed as a percentage of this baseline response. Horizontal line in each panel designates the point of 50% blockade of baseline suppression (IC_{50}). For all drugs but κ-bungarotoxin, each set of means is based on $N = 5$ animals; for κ-bungarotoxin, $N = 2$ animals. (From Kujawa et al., 1994a, with permission.)

appear to have an unusual pharmacology: it was readily blocked by strychnine and by ACh antagonists. The drugs active at the neuromuscular junction (nicotinic, Nm, e.g., curare) were more potent than those active at autonomic ganglia (nicotinic, Nn, e.g., trimethaphan) or at smooth muscle (muscarinic, M, e.g., atropine). Kujawa et al. added another unusual property of the receptor: a block by the GABA receptor antagonist, bicuculline. Again because of the complexity of the preparation, each drug's exact site of action remains obscure, but the unusual pharmacology obtained with electrical stimulation was confirmed utilizing natural stimulation of the MOC nerve fibers.

Antagonists—in Vitro

Housley and Ashmore (1991) were the first to demonstrate that the ACh receptor protein's spectrum of pharmacology to ACh antagonists at the level of the isolated OHC was similar to that obtained using the whole animal (Figure 2–8; potency in blocking applied ACH: curare > strychnine > atropine > pirenzepine). Fuchs and Murrow (1992b) demonstrated a similar spectrum of pharmacological activity in the chick hair cells (Figure 2–9; potency: strychnine > timethaphan > curare > atropine). Kakeha-

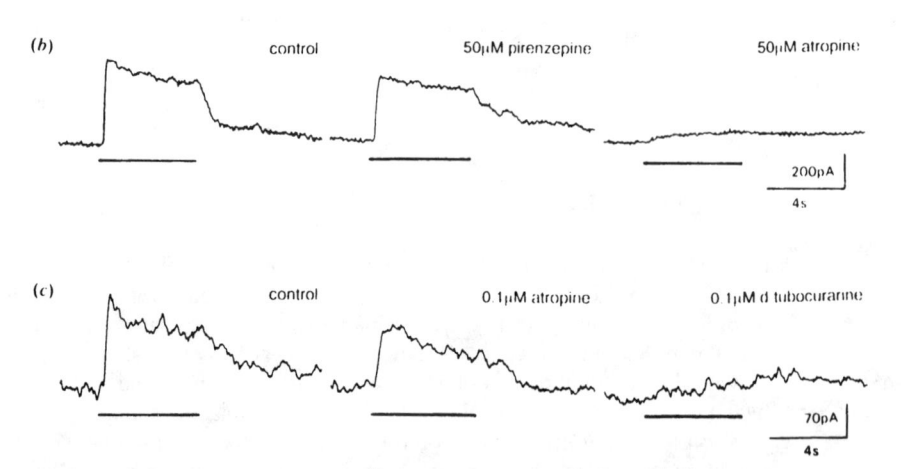

Figure 2–8. Localization and synaptic properties of the ACh response. (a) Not shown. (b) Atropine was more effective than pirenzipine as an antagonist when included at equimolar concentrations with 50 µM ACh. (c) The nicotinic antagonist d-tubocurarine was more effective than atropine when both were applied at 100 nM along with 50 µM ACh; 5 s pressure pulse monitored below. Holding potential, –50 mV in (a) -60 mV in (b, c). (From Housley and Ashmore, 1991, with permission.)

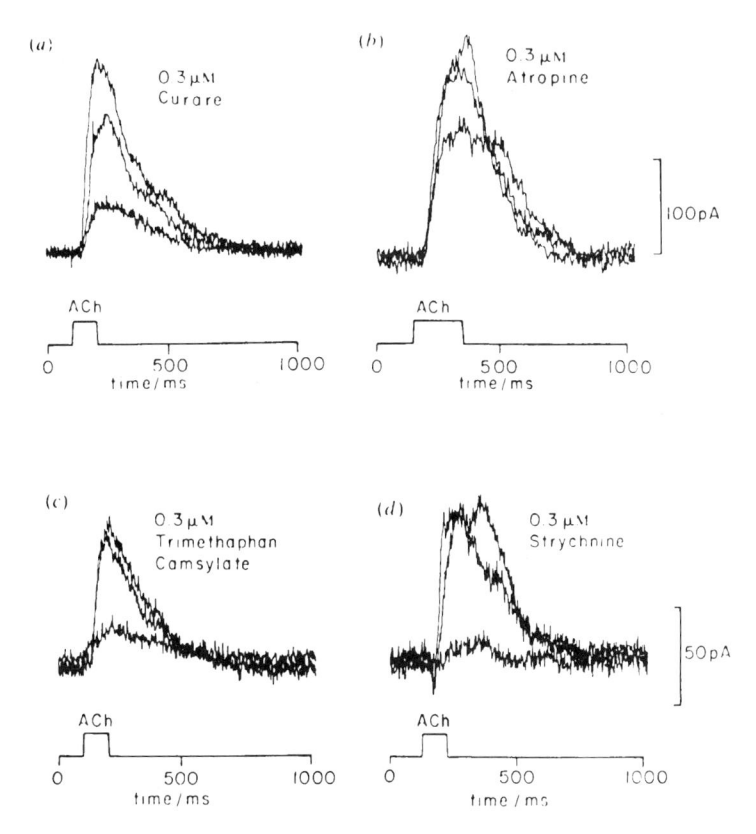

Figure 2–9. Antagonists of the hair cell ACh response. (a) Curare (0.3 μM) blocked 62% of the ACh (100 μM) response. Membrane potential –44 mV. (b) Atropine (0.3 μM) blocked 37% of the ACh response. Membrane potential –24 mV. (c) Trimethaphan camsylate (0.3 μM) blocked 77% of the ACh response. Membrane potential –54 mV. (d) Strychnine (0.3 μM) blocked 79% of the response. Membrane potential –54 mV. Application of ACh indicated by the lower bar. Pre- and post-controls shown in each panel. All antagonists were shown to be completely reversible in these or other cells. (From Fuchs and Murrow, 1992b, with permission.)

ta, Nakagawa, Takasaka, and Akaike (1993) tested muscarinic antagonists and found the following order of potency against applied ACh: atropine = 4-DAMP > AFDX 116 > pirenzepine. Erostegui, Norris, and Bobbin (1994) compared many of the drugs in the same preparation, extending the previous findings and showing that bicuculline blocks the effect of applied ACh (Figure 2–10; Table 2–2). Overall, the data of Erostegui et al. indicate the following order of potency of antagonists against applied ACh: strychnine, a glycine receptor antagonist > curare, a

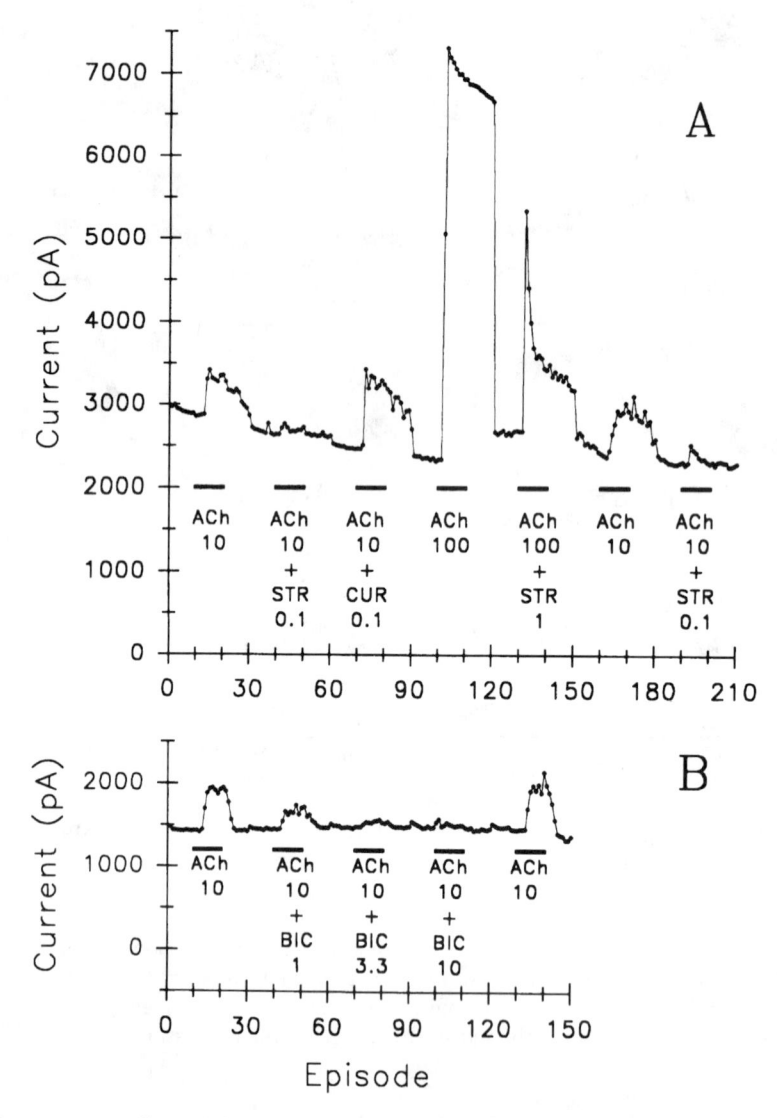

Figure 2–10. Effect of the nontraditional cholinergic antagonists, strychnine (STR) and bicuculline (BIC) on the response to ACh. A: strychnine (0.1 μM) blocked ACh. The large response (4.7 nA) to ACh (100 μM) is suppressed in great extent by strychnine at 1 μM. Bicuculline (3.3 and 10 μM) blocked ACh. Numbers near the drug abbreviations are drug concentrations in μM. Shown are data obtained as voltage clamp current responses at zero mV utilizing the same step protocol as illustrated and described in Figure 2–2. See Figure 2–2 for further description. (From Erostegui et al., 1994, with permission.)

TABLE 2–2. Summary of effects of ACh antagonists on the ACh evoked current response in isolated OHCs.

ACh Antagonist	Concentration (in millimolar):								
	0.1	0.3	1	3.3	10	33	100	330	1000
Curare	0%	–	87%	100%					
Trimethaphan Camsylate	0%	–	40%	100%	100%				
α-bungarotoxin	0%	0%	50%	100%					
Atropine	–	–	0%	45%	100%	100%			
4-DAMP	–	–	0%	25%	66%	100%			
AFDX	–	–	–	0%	44%	100%			
Pirenzepine	–	–	–	–	–	–	50%	100%	100%
Strychnine	75%	–	100%						
Bicuculline	–	–	75%	90%	100%				

Source: Erostegui et al. (1994).

Note: Shown are the concentrations of antagonist (millimolar) tested against the current induced by 10 μM ACh in single isolated OHCs. Percentage indicates the number of cells in which the induced current was blocked out of the number of cells tested with the concentration of antagonist.

Nm receptor antagonist > bicuculline, a GABA receptor antagonist > atropine, a M receptor antagonist. Surprisingly, the pharmacological data obtained in vivo matched fairly closely with the data obtained in vitro. Because these studies used single cells and studied the blockade of applied ACh, the drugs were all acting at the OHC membrane, probably at the ACh receptor protein. However, even single cell experiments are complex; some of the drugs that blocked the action of applied ACh may have been acting at ion channels or other sites on the OHC and not directly on the OHC receptor protein. More studies will have to be done to prove the site of action.

Agonists–in Vivo

The use of antagonists characterizes a receptor protein to a certain extent. On the other hand, agonists can give more information, as these are the chemicals that activate the receptor protein to initiate subsequent cellular events. For instance, when ACh was combined with eserine (which blocked cholinesterase from degrading the ACh molecule) and placed into the cochlear fluids, it not only mimicked the effects of efferent stimulation, but in the face of the continuous application of ACh the response declined or desensitized while concurrently the efferents became ineffective (Bobbin & Konishi, 1971a, 1971b; Figure 2–11). Kujawa, Glattke, Fallon, and Bobbin (1992) replicated this earlier work by utilizing DPOAEs and again demonstrated desensitization. These studies demonstrated that ACh could act at this synapse in a manner similar to activation of the MOC efferent fibers. In addition, they demonstrated desensitization of the response and emphasized the activity of cholinesterase in destroying applied acetylcholine. More importantly for this discussion, Konishi and I demonstrated that neither nicotine, a powerful agonist at the nicotinic receptors, nor arecoline, an agonist at muscarinic receptors, had much of an effect (Bobbin & Konishi, 1971a, 1974). Galley et al. (1973) described

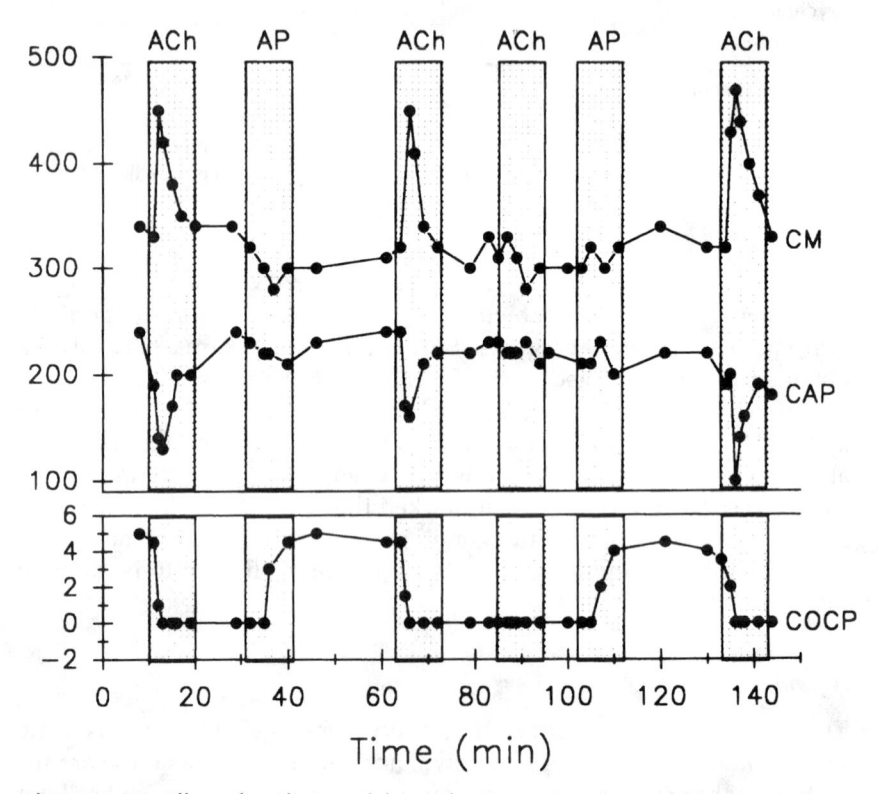

Figure 2–11. Effect of perfusion of the scala tympani on the cochlear microphonic (CM) (600 Hz, 64 dB SPL) and auditory nerve potential (AP) (6 kHz, 81 dB SPL) recorded without COCB stimulation, and the slow potential change (COCP) elicited by COCB stimulation. The scala tympani was perfused with artificial perilymph (A) and with acetylcholine chloride (250 μM) together with eserine sulphate (10 μM; B). (From Bobbin and Konishi, 1971b, with permission.)

the low potency of the muscarinic agonist, muscarone. Thus, even though the data with antagonists demonstrated the receptor was nicotinic (i.e., Nn), the data with agonists suggested the receptor was not nicotinic or muscarinic as the agonists had no effect.

Agonists–in Vitro

Recently, Kakehata et al. (1993) confirmed the in vivo data utilizing individual isolated OHCs. They demonstrated very little or no activity with nicotine, muscarine, McN-A-343, oxotremorine, and oxotremorine-M (Figure 2–12). They found that the most potent agonists were acetylcholine and carbachol. Erostegui et al. (1994) found that not only were nicotine and muscarine ineffective, but so was cytisine (Figure 2–13). On the other hand, Erostegui et al. found that DMPP and suberyldicholine, additional nicotinic agonists, were active.

Table 2–3 summarizes the unique pharmacology of this unusual receptor. The ACh receptor protein appears to have an unusual spectrum of activity in response to the various antagonists; the antagonists listed in Table 2–1 all block the ACh receptor on OHCs even though they are specific for the other receptors listed (e.g., pirenzepine vs the M1 receptor). In addition, the receptor fails to be activated by either the M receptor agonist, muscarine, or the Nn and Nm receptor agonist, nicotine. Cytisine, an additional nicotinic receptor agonist also failed to activate the receptor. On the other hand, it was activated by DMPP and suberyldicholine. To the best of our knowledge, no receptor to date has been described with this spectrum of pharmacological activity (e.g., Seguela, Wadiche, Dineley-Miller, Dani, & Patrick, 1993), although recent results with an alpha 9 receptor subunit come very close (Elgoyhen, Johnson, Boulter, Vetter, & Heinemann, 1994). So it appears that the receptor protein on the OHCs may be unique and not described to date.

In previous publications, I argued that the receptor was nicotinic, but this was based on the pharmacology to the antagonists. On the other hand, it is difficult to name it nicotinic when nicotine has no effect. In general, receptors are named after the drug most active at the receptor, for example, nicotinic or muscarinic. So it seems then that the ACh receptor on the OHC should not be called nicotinic or muscarinic. As suberyldicholine is one of the most potent agonists, the receptor should be called a suberyldicholinic receptor, or "subdic" for short (Bobbin, 1994).

Receptors have been grouped into families based on their molecular configuration. For instance, at present ACh receptors are classified as belonging either to the nicotinic family or the muscarinic family. At present we do not know to which family the ACh receptor on the OHC

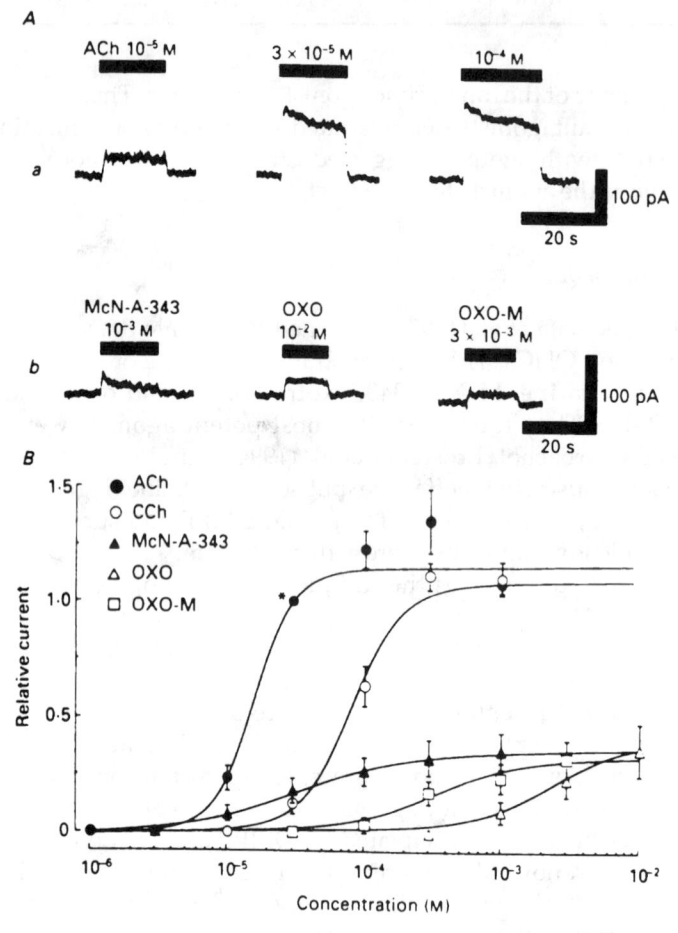

Figure 2–12. I_{ACh} in dissociated outer hair cells (OHCs). A a, I_{ACh} at various concentrations under voltage-clamp conditions using the perforated patch-clamp technique. The holding potential (V_H) was –40 mV. Horizontal bars above each response indicate a period of continuous ACh application. The current was recorded from a 40 μm OHC of the second turn. The resting membrane potential (VR) and the input impedance were –60 mV and 33 MΩ, respectively. The amplitude of the current injected to hold the membrane potential of –40 mV was 600 pA. A b, representative current induced by McN-A-343, oxotremorine (OXO), and oxotremorine-M (OXO-M). The 50 μm cell was obtained from the second turn. The V_R and the input impedance were –62 mV and 67 MΩ, respectively. The amplitude of the current injected to hold the membrane potential of –40 mV was 320 pA. B, concentration-response relationships for ACh, carbamylcholine (Cch), and various muscarinic agonists. Amplitudes of currents induced by each drug at various concentrations were normalized to the current induced by 3×10^{-5} M ACh (*). Each point is the mean ± S.E.M. of four to seven cells. (From Kakehata et al., 1993, with permission.)

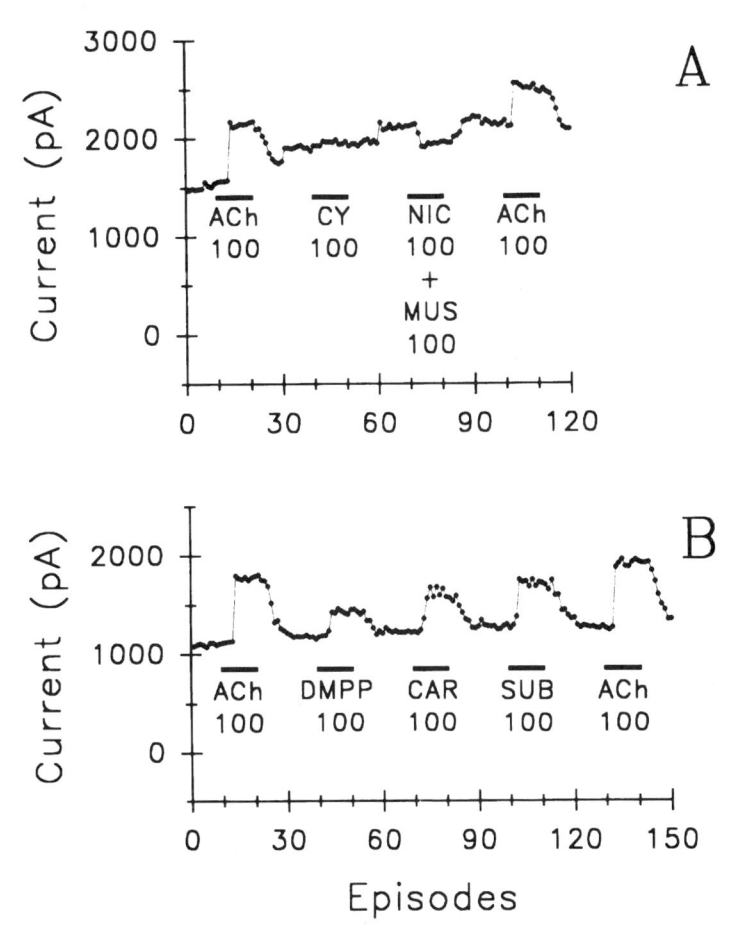

Figure 2–13. Effect of the ACh receptor agonists compared to ACh in two cells; frame **A**, cytisine (CY) and nicotine with muscarine (NIC + MUS); frame **B**: DMPP, carbachol (CAR) and suberyldicholine (SUB). In frame **A** between records (every 30 episodes) an apparent recovery of some current strength occurred as in Figure 2–8. Note the mixture of nicotine with muscarine suppressed the current. Numbers near the drug abbreviation are drug concentrations in μM. Shown are data obtained as voltage clamp current responses at zero mV utilizing the same step protocol as illustrated and described in Figure 2–2. See Figure 2–2 for further description. (From Erostegui et al., 1994, with permission.)

TABLE 2–3. Summary of the various antagonists of ACh at the OHC and a list of the other receptors where these antagonists are thought to be most selective.

Receptor Type[a]	Agonist	Location	ACh Antagonist[b]
suberyldicholine or subdic (S)	Ach, suberyl-dicholine	OHCs	strychnine
nicotonic (Nm)	ACh, nicotine	skeletal muscle	curare, α-BTX
nicotinic (Nn)	ACh, nicotine	autonomic ganglia	trimethaphan
muscarinic (M)	ACh, muscarine	smooth muscle glands	atropine
muscarinic (M_1)	ACh, muscarine	"	pirenzepine
muscarinic (M_2)	ACh, muscarine	"	AF-DX 116
muscarinic (M_3)	ACh, muscarine	"	4-DAMP
glycinergic (gly)	glycine	central nervous system	strychnine
GABAergic (GABA)	GABA	"	bicuculline

[a]Suberyldicholine is the name proposed for the ACh receptor type on the OHCs.
[b]All of the antagonists listed block the effects of ACh at the OHC. Only strychnine is listed at the OHC because it is the most potent antagonist against ACh.

belongs. It is unlikely that ACh belongs to a new family, even though new families of receptors are being discovered (e.g., ATP family; Valera et al., 1994). However, until the molecular composition of the subdic receptor is determined, the "family" will remain unknown.

Adenosine triphosphate (ATP)

ATP was first suggested to be a candidate for a neurotransmitter or neuromodulator in the cochlea based on its relative potency in reducing the compound action potential of the auditory nerve (Bobbin & Thompson, 1978). Subsequent studies have demonstrated that ATP increases intracellular Ca^{2+} levels in inner hair cells (Dulon, Mollard, & Aran 1991) and Deiters cells (Dulon et al., 1993) and has powerful effects on the membrane potential of the OHCs (Ashmore & Ohmori, 1990; Housley, Greenwood, & Ashmore, 1992; Kakehata et al., 1993; Kujawa, Erostegui, Fallon,

Crist, & Bobbin, 1994b; Nakagawa, Akaike, Kimitsuki, Komune, & Arima, 1990). ATP activates a receptor on OHCs that induces a large inward current and so depolarizes the OHC.

ATP is metabolized very rapidly to adenosine, a compound with little activity in the cochlea. However, chemists have made a few ATP analogues that are not as rapidly metabolized, such as ATP-γ-S. Recently, Kujawa et al. (1994b) demonstrated that ATP-γ-S was one of the most potent compounds studied when instilled into the perilymph: ATP-γ-S abolished the CAP and the DPOAEs, and decreased the low intensity sound-evoked SP while it increased the high intensity sound-evoked SP (Figure 2–14). In addition, Kujawa, Fallon, and Bobbin (1994c) demonstrated powerful effects of ATP antagonists on cochlear potentials suggesting a role for endogenously released ATP in normal physiology.

The role of ATP and its receptor proteins in the cochlea is unknown. It may have both a paracrine and an autocrine role. Some suggest ATP is released from the efferent nerve fibers and as such is utilized as a depolarizing agent to counter the hyperpolarizing effects of ACh. Others suggest it may be acting on the scala media side of the OHC (near the stereocilia) to regulate the polarization of the OHC (Housley et al., 1992). In addition, ATP may have a role in programmed cell death (Valera, Hussy, Evans, Adami, North, Surprenant, & Buell, 1994). In summary, ATP has powerful effects in the cochlea, but the role of these effects in the physiology of the cochlea remains to be determined.

Other chemicals

GABA appears to be a transmitter at a small number of efferent nerve fibers that synapse on OHCs (see review by Eybalin, 1993). GABA may allow ions such as chloride to enter the cell and so hyperpolarizes the OHC (Gitter & Zenner, 1992).

Additional chemicals have been suggested to have a possible role at the OHCs. Glutamate, which is the transmitter between IHCs and the afferent nerves, and probably the transmitter between the OHCs and their afferent nerves (Bobbin, 1991) when applied acutely has no effect on the currents recorded from the OHCs in the whole cell voltage clamp configuration (Chen & Bobbin, 1994). However, glutamate may have a role on second messenger chemicals inside the OHCs that we cannot detect by measuring acute changes in cell current. Calcitonin-gene-related-peptide (CGRP) is another chemical found in the efferents innervating the OHCs for which a role has yet to be determined (Eybalin, 1993).

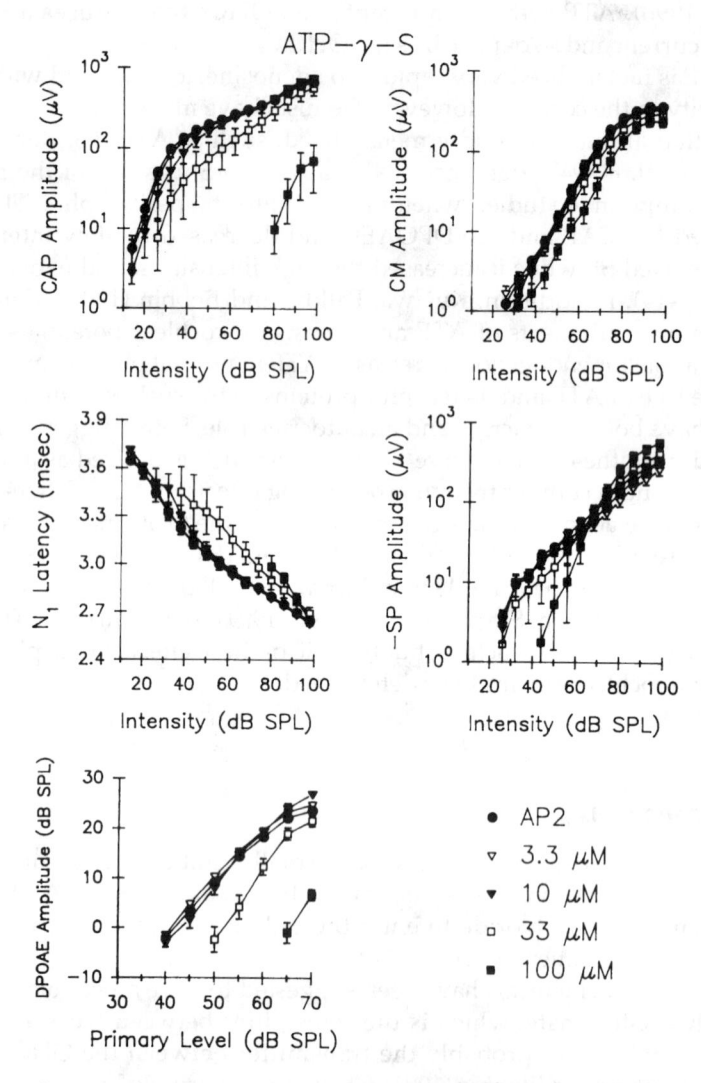

Figure 2–14. Effect of ATP-γ-S on CAP, N1 latency, SP, CM, and DPOAE responses as a function of stimulus intensity. Shown are functions recorded after pre-drug artificial perilymph perfusion No. 2 (AP2) and after perfusion with increasing concentrations (3.3–100 μM) of ATP-γ-S. Data are represented as means ± S.E. across 5 animals. (From Kujawa et al., 1994b, with permission.)

RECEPTOR MECHANISMS

The action of these chemicals at the level of the OHC is summarized in Figure 2–15. The movement of the stereocilia opens the transduction channel allowing potassium ions into the cell which results in depolarization of the OHC (see review by Roberts, Howard, & Hudspeth, 1988). This activates the motor protein in the OHC membrane that causes the

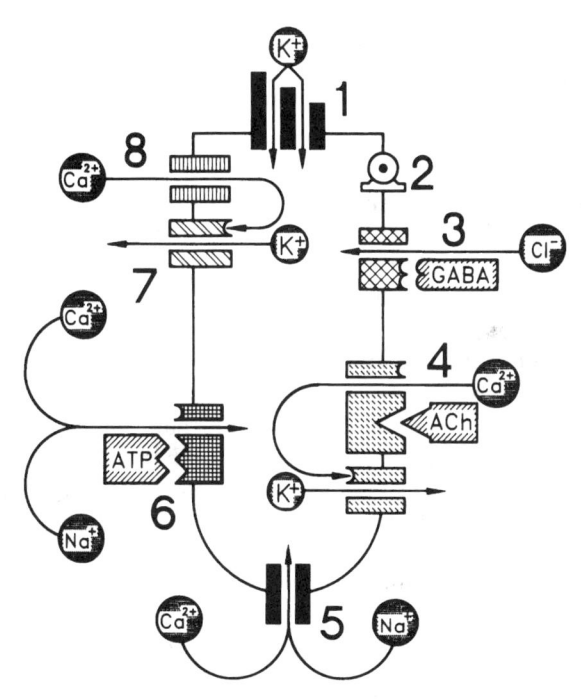

1. transduction channel
2. motor
3. GABA–receptor & ion channel complex
4. ACh–receptor & ion channel complex
5. non–specific cation channel
6. ATP–receptor & ion channel complex
7. K_{Ca} and K_n channel
8. L–type Ca^{2+} channel

Figure 2–15. Model of an OHC illustrating the various ion channel proteins in the membrane and available to alter the membrane potential.

length change in the cell, the motor being sensitive to the voltage of the cell (depolarization or voltage change in a positive direction = decrease in length; hyperpolarization or voltage change in a negative direction = increase in length).

In Figure 2–15 I have represented three types of ion channels that will respond to voltage changes in the cell: a nonspecific cation channel, an L-type Ca^{2+} channel, and at least two types of Ca^{2+}-activated potassium channels which are represented in Figure 2–14 as one channel (Housley & Ashmore, 1992; Nakagawa et al., 1991). These ion channels are voltage-activated channels, that is, they will open in response to voltage changes and allow certain ions to move across the membrane of the OHC. The ion flows they allow will in turn change the voltage of the cell. GABA, ACh, and ATP, which are called "ligands," act on receptor proteins that regulate or open other ion channels and, therefore, these channels are called "ligand-gated channels." Ligand-gated channels are usually not opened by voltage changes. Ligands can act on the receptor protein which is an actual part of the ion channel or they can act on receptor proteins that interact with G proteins, which in turn can act on ion channels and other enzymes in the cell. In the latter case the mechanism of receptor action is called metabotropic and in the former case it is called ionotropic.

Whether the subdic receptor protein is metabotropic or ionotropic is currently being debated. As mentioned previously, Housley and Ashmore were the first to demonstrate that, in mammalian cochlear OHCs, ACh induces an opening of a channel (K_{ACh}) that allows K^+ ions to move across the membrane of the OHC, down its electrical and chemical gradient. At membrane potentials positive to –70 mV, K^+ will move out of the OHC and result in a hyperpolarization of the cell. Experimentally, the opening of the K_{ACh} channel induced by ACh requires the presence of both extracellular and intracellular free Ca^{2+}. Therefore, most researchers feel that the opening of the K_{ACh} channel by ACh involves an intermediate step which increases the level of free Ca^{2+} inside the cell adjacent to the K_{ACh} channel. This intermediate step may consist of ACh directly opening an ion channel linked to the receptor that allows Ca^{2+} to enter the cell, as illustrated in the Figure 2–15 (Fuchs & Murrow, 1992a). In contrast, Kakehata et al. (1993) suggest that ACh stimulates phosphatidylinositol metabolism via a PTX-sensitive G-protein. The phosphatidylinositol then releases Ca^{2+} from intracellular stores to act on the KACh channel. Such a mechanism is illustrated in Figure 2–16. So the major immediate question that needs to be answered is what is the mechanism of the subdic receptor: Does the receptor act by opening a Ca^{2+}-selective cation channel (ionotropic) or does it activate a G protein (metabotropic)?

In the OHCs, ATP appears to open a cation selective channel to allow sodium and Ca^{2+} into the cell (depolarization) as shown in Figure 2–15.

Others suggest that ATP may also activate the G-protein coupled to the phosphoinositol cascade in a manner similar to ACh, as shown in Figure 2–16 (Niedzielski & Schacht, 1992).

GABA appears to open an ion channel permeable to the chloride ion. This would hyperpolarize the cell similar to the effects of acetylcholine.

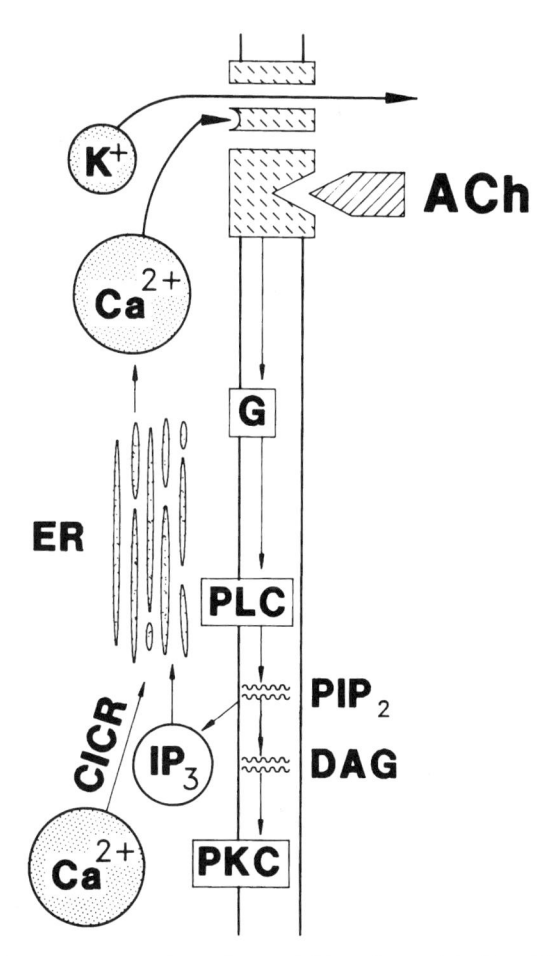

Figure 2–16. An alternative model (metabotropic) of the ACh receptor\ion channel complex illustrating a possible role for G protein and ionositol triphosphate (IP$_3$) in providing the intracellular Ca^{2+} for opening the K$^+$ channel. G: g protein; PLC: phospholipase C; PIP$_2$: phosphoinositol bisphosphate; DAG: diacylglycerol; PKC: phosphokinase C; CICR: calcium-induced calcium release; ER: endoplasmic reticulum.

In summary, these voltage-sensitive and ligand-activated channels in concert or alone can modify the voltage of the cell and the cells' length and length-change response to sound. In this manner, the active process is regulated and modulated. When and how all these channels are orchestrated to yield a functional active process awaits additional research.

Acknowledgments: The author wishes to thank Maureen Fallon and Jim Bolongaro for drawing the illustrations and Anastas Nenov, Chu Chen, Latasha Bright, Elaine McDonald, Cristopher LeBlanc, and Ruth Skellett for help. This work was funded in part by the following: NIH research grants DC00722, DC00379, and DAMD 17-93-V-3013, Kam's Fund for Hearing Research, and the Louisiana Lions Eye Foundation.

GLOSSARY

Autocrine. A chemical substance, also known as messenger, that is released from cells and reaches targets (receptors) located on the same cell by diffusion, for example, autoneurotransmitters.

Depolarization. Change in the resting membrane potential of a cell in the positive direction, less negative.

Hyperpolarization. Change in the resting membrane potential of a cell in the negative direction, less positive.

Ionotropic. A receptor mechanism for a neurotransmitter: the receptor protein is part of an ion channel\receptor protein complex and opens or closes the ion channel directly in response to the presence of a ligand (i.e., any compound that binds to a receptor) for that receptor.

Metabotropic. A receptor mechanism for a neurotransmitter: the receptor protein acts via another protein such as a g protein to activate or inhibit enzymes and possibly open, close, or modify ion channels.

Muscarinic receptor protein. The receptor activated by the neurotransmitter, acetylcholine (ACh), and the drug, muscarine, located at the autonomic innervation of glands, cardiac muscle, and smooth muscle—abbreviated M.

Neurotransmitter. Chemical released from a sensory receptor cell or nerve cell on depolarization of that cell. On release the chemical diffuses across the gap between the releasing cell and an adjoining cell to act on the adjoining cell to induce a change in its electrical or chemical properties.

Nicotinic receptor protein. The receptor activated by the neurotransmitter, acetylcholine (ACh), and by the drug, nicotine, located at the neuromuscular junction of skeletal muscle—abbreviated Nm.

Paracrine. A chemical substance, also known as a messenger, that is released from cells and reaches different target cells by diffusion, for example, neurotransmitters.

Receptor protein. Protein in the membrane of a cell that accepts a chemical messenger (ligand) such as the neurotransmitter, changes its configuration on accepting the neurotransmitter, and so induces subsequent reactions in the cell, such as opening of an ion channel to allow for diffusion of that ion down its concentration and electrical gradient.

REFERENCES

Ashmore, J. F., & Ohmori, H. (1990). Control of intracellular calcium by ATP in isolated outer hair cells of the guinea-pig cochlea. *Journal of Physiology, 428,* 109–131.

Bledsoe, S. C., Jr., Bobbin, R. P., & Puel, J.-L. (1988). Neurotransmission in the inner ear. In A. F. Jahn, & J. R. Santos-Sacchi (Eds.), *Physiology of hearing* (pp. 385–406). New York: Raven Press.

Bobbin, R. P. (1991). Cochlear chemical neurotransmission. In *Encyclopedia of human biology* (Vol. 2, pp. 521–525). San Diego, CA: Academic Press.

Bobbin, R. P. (1994, September). *Cholinergic pharmacology of medial efferent regulation of the active mechanisms.* Paper presented at the First International Inner Ear Neuropharmacology Symposium, Montpellier, France.

Bobbin, R. P., & Konishi, T. (1971a). Action of some cholinomimetics and cholinolytics on the effect of the crossed olivocochlear bundle (COCB). *Journal of the Acoustical Society of America, 49,* 122.

Bobbin, R. P., & Konishi, T. (1971b). Acetylcholine mimics crossed olivocochlear bundle stimulation. *National New Biology, 231,* 222–223.

Bobbin, R. P., & Konishi, T. (1974). Action of cholinergic and anticholinergic drugs at the crossed olivocochlear bundle-hair cell junction. *Acta Otolaryngologica 77,* 56–65.

Bobbin, R. P., & Thompson, M. H. (1978). Effects of putative transmitters on afferent cochlear transmission. *Annals of Otology, Rhinology, and Laryngology 87,* 185-190.

Churchill, J. A., Schuknecht, H. P., & Doran, R. (1956). Acetylcholinesterase activity in the cochlea. *Laryngoscope, 66,* 1–15.

Daigneault, E. A. (1981). Pharmacology of cochlear efferents. In R. D. Brown & E. A. Daigneault (Eds.), *Pharmacology of hearing* (pp. 231–270). New York: John Wiley & Sons.

Desmedt, J. E., & Monaco, P. (1960). Suppression by strychnine of the efferent inhibitory effect induced by the olivocochlear bundle. *Archives of International Pharmacodyn, 129,* 244–248.

Dulon, D. (1994). Ca^{2+} signaling in Deiters cells of the guinea-pig cochlea active process in supporting cells? In A. Flock (Ed.), *Active hearing* (pp. 195–207). New York: Elsevier Science.

Dulon, D., Blanchet, C., & Laffon, E. (1994). Photo-released intracellular Ca^{2+} evokes reversible mechanical responses in supporting cells of the guinea-pig organ of Corti. *Biochemistry and Biophysical Research Community 201*, 1263–1269.

Dulon, D., Moataz, R., & Mollard, P. (1993). Characterization of Ca^{2+} signals generated by extracellular nucleotides in supporting cells of the organ of Corti. *Cell Calcium, 14*, 245–254.

Dulon, D., Mollard, P., & Aran, J.-M (1991). Extracellular ATP elevates cytosolic Ca^{2+} in cochlear inner hair cells. *NeuroReport, 2*, 69–72.

Elgoyhen, A. B., Johnson, D. S., Boulter, J., Vetter, D. E., & Heinemann, S. (1994). α 9: An acetylcholine receptor with novel pharmacological properties expressed in rat cochlear hair cells. *Cell, 79*, 705–715.

Erostegui, C., Norris, C. H., & Bobbin, R. P. (1994). In vitro pharmacologic characterization of a cholinergic receptor on outer hair cells. *Hearing Research, 74*, 135–147.

Eybalin, M. (1993). Neurotransmitters and neuromodulators of the mammalian cochlea. *Physiological Reviews, 73*, 309–373.

Fex, J. (1968). Efferent inhibition in the cochlea by the olivocochlear bundle. In A. V. S. DeReuck & J. Knight (Eds.), *Ciba Foundation symposium on hearing mechanisms in vertebrates* (pp. 169–186). Boston: Little, Brown.

Fex, J., & Adams, J. C. (1978). α-Bungarotoxin blocks reversibly cholinergic inhibition in the cochlea. *Brain Research 159*, 440–444.

Fuchs, P. A., & Murrow, B. W. (1992a). Cholinergic inhibition of short (outer) hair cells of the chick's cochlea. *Journal of Neuroscience, 12*, 800–809.

Fuchs, P. A., & Murrow, B. W. (1992b). A novel cholinergic receptor mediates inhibition of chick cochlear hair cells. *Proceedings of the Royal Society of London, (B) 248*, 35–40.

Galley, N., Klinke, R., Oertel, W., Pause, M., & Storch, W.-H. (1973). The effect of intracochlearly administered acetylcholine-blocking agents on the efferent synapses of the cochlea. *Brain Research, 64*, 55–63.

Gitter, A. H., & Zenner, H. P. (1992). Gamma-aminobutyric acid receptor activation of outer hair cells in the guinea pig cochlea. *European Archives of Otorhinolaryngology, 249*, 62–65.

Guth, P. S., Norris, C. H., & Bobbin, R. P. (1976). The pharmacology of transmission in the peripheral auditory system. *Pharmacology Review, 28*, 95–125.

Housley, G. D., & Ashmore, J. F. (1991). Direct measurement of the action of acetylcholine on isolated outer hair cells of the guinea pig cochlea. *Proceedings of the Royal Society of London, (B) 244*, 161–167.

Housley, G. D., & Ashmore, J. F. (1992). Ionic currents of outer hair cells isolated from guinea-pig cochlea. *Journal of Physiology, 448*, 73–98.

Housley, G. D., Greenwood, D., & Ashmore, J. F. (1992). Localization of cholinergic and purinergic receptors on outer hair cells isolated from the guinea-pig cochlea. *Proceedings of the Royal Society of London, (B) 249*, 265–273.

Kakehata, S., Nakagawa, T., Takasaka, T., & Akaike, N. (1993). Cellular mechanism of acetylcholine-induced response in dissociated outer hair cells of guinea-pig cochlea. *Journal of Physiology, 463*, 227–244.

Kujawa, S. G., Glattke, T. J., Fallon, M., & Bobbin, R. P. (1992). Intracochlear application of acetylcholine alters sound-induced mechanical events within the cochlear partition. *Hearing Research, 61*, 106–116.

Kujawa, S. G., Glattke, T. J., Fallon, M., & Bobbin, R. P. (1993). Contralateral sound suppresses distortion product otoacoustic emissions through cholinergic mechanisms. *Hearing Research, 68*, 97–106.

Kujawa, S. G., Glattke, T. J., Fallon, M., & Bobbin, R. P. (1994a). A nicotinic-like receptor mediates suppression of distortion product otoacoustic emissions by contralateral sound. *Hearing Research, 74*, 122–134.

Kujawa, S. G., Erostegui, C., Fallon, M., Crist, J., & Bobbin, R. P. (1994b). Effects of Adenosine 5'-triphosphate and related agonists on cochlear function. *Hearing Research, 76*, 87–100.

Kujawa, S. G., Fallon, M., & Bobbin, R. P. (1994c). ATP antagonists cibacron blue, basilen blue and suramin alter sound-evoked responses of the cochlea and auditory nerve. *Hearing Research, 78*, 181–188.

Liberman, M. C., & Kawase, T. (1992). Anti-masking effects of the cochlear efferent bundle. *Proceedings of the Sendai Symposium, 2*, 67–71.

Moataz, R., Saito, T., & Dulon, D. (1992). Evidence for voltage sensitive Ca^{2+} channels in supporting cells of the organ of Corti: Characterization by indo-1 fluorescence. *Advances in the Biosciences, 83*, 53–59.

Nakagawa, T., Akaike, N., Kimitsuki, T., Komune, S., & Arima, T. (1990). ATP-induced current in isolated outer hair cells of guinea pig cochlea. *Journal of Neurophysiology, 63*, 1068–1074.

Nakagawa, T., Kakehata, S., Akaike, N., Komune, S., Takasaka, T., & Uemura, T. (1991). Calcium channel in isolated outer hair cells of guinea pig cochlea. *Neuroscience Letters, 125*, 81–84.

Niedzielski, A. S., & Schacht, J. (1992). P_2 purinoceptors stimulate inositol phosphate release in the organ of Corti. *NeuroReport, 3*, 273–275.

Puel, J.-L., & Rebillard, G. (1990). Effect of contralateral sound stimulation on the distortion product 2F1-F2: Evidence that the medial efferent system is involved. *Journal of the Acoustical Society of America, 87*, 1630–1635.

Pujol, R. (1990). Cochlear physiology and physiopathology. Recent data. *Drugs of Today, 26*, 43–57.

Roberts, W. M., Howard, J., & Hudspeth, A. J. (1988). Hair cells: Transduction, tuning, and transmission in the inner ear. *Annals Review of Cell Biology, 4*, 63–92.

Santos-Sacchi, J., & Dilger, D. P. (1988). Whole-cell currents and mechanical responses of isolated outer hair cells. *Hearing Research, 35*, 143–150.

Schuknecht, H. F., Churchill, J. A., & Doran, R. (1959). The localization of acetylcholinesterase in the cochlea. *Archive of Otolaryngology, 69*, 549–559.

Seguela, P., Wadiche, J., Dineley-Miller, K., Dani, J. A., & Patrick, J. W. (1993). Molecular cloning, functional properties, and distribution of rat brain α_7: A nicotinic cation channel highly permeable to calcium. *Journal of Neurosciences, 13*, 596–604.

Valera, S., Hussy, N., Evans, R. J., Adami, N., North, R. A., Surprenant, A., & Buell, G. (1994). A new class of ligand-gated ion channel defined by P_{2x} receptor for extracellular ATP. *Nature, 371*, 516–519.

Warr, W. B., & Guinan, J. J. (1979). Efferent innervation of the organ of Corti: Two separate systems. *Brain Research, 173*, 152–155.

3

Suppression of Otoacoustic Emissions in Normal Hearing Individuals

Linda J. Hood, Ph.D.
Charles I. Berlin, Ph.D.
Annette Hurley, M.S.
Han Wen, M.S.B.E.

Kresge Hearing Research Laboratory of the South,
Department of Otorhinolaryngology and Biocommunication,
Louisiana State University Medical Center
New Orleans, Louisiana

INTRODUCTION

The recent discoveries of evoked otoacoustic emissions (Kemp, 1978) and of outer hair cell motility (Brownell, Bader, Bertrand, & deRibaupierre, 1985) have contributed to a significant increase in the understanding of the role of cochlear micromechanics in the processing of auditory stimuli. Otoacoustic emissions are low-level sounds that emanate from the cochlea and can be recorded from the external ear canal using sensitive low-noise microphones. They are associated with nonlinear processes present in the normal cochlea and enhanced sensitivity and tuning of the auditory system. The origin of otoacoustic emissions is ascribed to processes associated with the mechanical motion of the outer hair cells, thought to be controlled through the efferent auditory pathways via the olivocochlear system (Kemp, 1978; Kemp & Chum, 1980; Probst, Lonsbury-Martin, 1991; Norton & Widin, 1990).

There are two broad categories of otoacoustic emissions (OAEs): spontaneous and evoked (Table 3–1). Spontaneous otoacoustic emissions, or SOAEs, by definition occur spontaneously, requiring no external stim-

TABLE 3–1. Classification of otoacoustic emissions.

Category	Type	Stimulus
Spontaneous		None
Evoked	Transient	Clicks or tonebursts
	Distortion Product	Pairs of pure tones
	Stimulus Frequency	Swept pure tones

ulus to elicit a response. In contrast, evoked emissions fall into three classes, each requiring a different type of external stimulus. Transient evoked otoacoustic emissions (TEOAEs) are obtained in response to brief stimuli such as clicks or tonebursts, distortion product otoacoustic emissions (DPOAEs or DPEs) are produced by pairs of pure tones, and stimulus frequency emissions (SFOAEs) are generated by presentation of continuous tonal stimuli. Otoacoustic emissions have received extensive attention in human and animal research and several reviews are available (e.g., Glattke & Kujawa, 1991; Martin, Probst, & Lonsbury-Martin, 1990; Probst et al., 1991). Clinical applications have focused on TEOAEs and DPOAEs in the evaluation of cochlear function, screening for hearing loss in newborns, and monitoring changes in auditory function.

Emissions are not only valuable in analyzing the integrity of individual ears; they can also be used to evaluate interactions between the two ears by studying emission suppression following presentation of additional stimuli to the same, opposite, or both ears. A number of studies have described suppression of spontaneous and transient emissions in humans by contralateral acoustic stimuli (Berlin, Hood, Cecola, Jackson, & Szabo, 1993a; Collet et al., 1990; Grose, 1983; Schloth & Zwicker, 1983; Mott, Norton, Neely, & Warr, 1989; Rabinowitz & Widen, 1984; Ryan, Kemp, & Hinchcliffe, 1991; Veuillet, Collet, & Duclaux, 1991). These suppression effects observed in humans are consistent with suppression of both cochlear emissions and auditory nerve activity observed in animals (e.g. Buno, 1978; Liberman, 1989; Mountain, 1980; Puel & Rebillard, 1990).

Anatomical and physiological evidence supports the interdependent function of the two ears mediated through the efferent neural pathways which link one side of the auditory system to the other side via the medial and lateral components of the olivocochlear system (Warr & Guinan, 1978; Warr, Guinan, & White, 1986). The medial olivocochlear components terminate primarily on the outer hair cells, whereas the lateral olivocochlear components terminate mainly on primary auditory neurons at the base of the inner hair cells. Outer hair cell activity is believed to be modified through the medial efferent connections. Function of these pathways can be studied objectively and noninvasively in animals and in humans using suppression of otoacoustic emissions.

Suppression of transient evoked otoacoustic emissions has been a subject of study at Kresge Hearing Research Laboratory for several years. Research has focused on understanding the physiology of suppression of emissions, definition of the normal characteristics of suppression, parametric study of stimulus and external factors that affect suppression, the development of methodology that leads to efficient and reliable recording and analysis of suppression, and delineation of clinical applications. In this chapter, we focus on the characteristics of suppression in individuals with normal auditory function and describe the effects of stimulus and noise characteristics on suppression and the definition of suppression effects through specialized analysis techniques. This chapter is followed by a companion chapter which describes clinical patients who show no suppression of emissions and discusses ways in which suppression information can be used in the management of hearing loss.

Subjects

Subjects participating in the following studies all had normal hearing in both ears, defined as thresholds of 15 dB HL or better for the frequency range of .25 through 8 kHz. Middle ear measures (tympanograms and ipsilateral and contralateral acoustic reflex thresholds) were within normal limits and subjects had no history of neurological abnormality.

General TEOAE Recording Methods

For the studies described here, transient-evoked otoacoustic emissions were obtained using an Otodynamics ILO88 otoacoustic emissions system. Stimuli were 80-microsecond clicks which were nonlinear in our early studies, but linear in more recent studies. Nonlinear click trains present three stimuli of like phase followed by a fourth stimulus both opposite in phase and 10 dB higher in intensity. This type of stimulus paradigm is desirable in general emissions test situations to reduce stimulus artifact while maintaining a quantifiable otoacoustic emission. However, use of nonlinear click trains affects the true amplitude of the emission and thus makes absolute quantification of suppression effects difficult. Thus, the use of linear clicks (all clicks of like phase) is both desirable and possible since lower intensity stimuli are generally used in suppression studies. Suppressor (masker) stimuli are generated either externally (when contralateral noise is presented simultaneously) or internally by the ILO88 system (in a forward masking paradigm). When externally generated, noise levels are continually monitored with a probe microphone.

Three control (without contralateral noise) and three experimental (with contralateral noise) test conditions are alternated and averaged separately for each subject prior to analysis in accordance with the method suggested by Collet et al. (1990). Averages of 260 click trains of 4 clicks each are obtained for a total of 1,040 stimuli per condition, unless otherwise noted. Responses are accepted when the stimulus stability exceeds 80% and the response reproducibility exceeds 70%. Stimulus stability represents a comparison of stimulus level recorded in the ear canal at the beginning of the test to the level of the stimulus monitored throughout the test acquisition period. Response reproducibility represents the correlation of averages of half of the sweeps which are stored in one computer buffer and the other half of the sweeps stored in another memory buffer. These two averages are acquired by interleaving sweeps between two computer memories during the acquisition of an emission. A typical evoked otoacoustic emission obtained from a female subject with normal hearing using the ILO88 System is shown in Figure 3–1. In this case, the overall amplitude of the emission is 12.9 dB and the response reproducibility is 98%. The stimuli were linear clicks which were monitored at

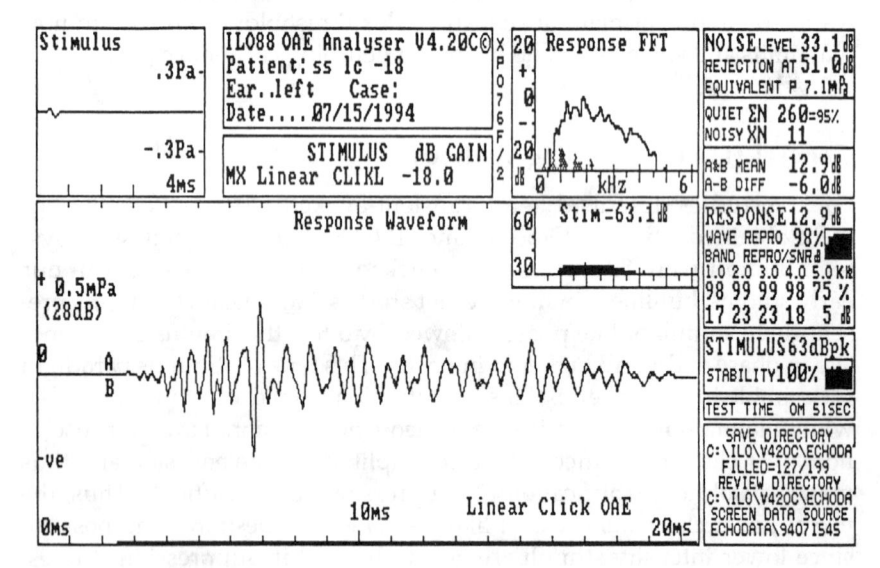

Figure 3–1. Transient Evoked Otoacoustic Emissions (TEOAEs) obtained from a normal subject using linear clicks.

an intensity of 63 dB peak sound pressure in the ear canal, and the stimulus stability during the test was 100%.

Early Studies

In our early studies of suppression, transient otoacoustic emissions were obtained using nonlinear clicks at 80 dB peak SP (sound pressure). The emissions were suppressed by either pure tones (at octave intervals from 250 to 4kHz), narrow band noises (centered at octave intervals from 250 to 4kHz), or broad band noise presented simultaneously to the contralateral ear. Results indicated greater suppression with increasing masker levels, greater effects with narrow-band noises than with pure tones, and greater suppression effects for lower frequency than higher frequency maskers. The details of these studies were reported in Berlin et al. (1993a).

In all of our studies, we reported suppression effects as dB differences in emission amplitude between conditions with and without noise rather than as equivalent dB, as Collet and colleagues have used (Collet et al., 1990; Veuillet et al., 1991). Although the differences observed in overall emission amplitude between conditions without and with noise appear small (on the order of 1 or 2 dB), they are quite consistent. We also observed that suppression effects are greater in certain time periods, which led us to the development of a method to analyze suppression of emissions in greater detail.

Development of Data Analysis Techniques

As we sought to refine our understanding of suppression, one of the authors (HW) developed an analysis program to quantify changes in transient evoked otoacoustic emissions obtained under varying test conditions (Wen, Berlin, Hood, Jackson, Hurley, 1993). The Kresge EchoMaster Program (current version 3.1) is compatible with the Otodynamics ILO88 file structure and allows detailed comparisons of root-mean-square (RMS) amplitude, cross correlations, and time delays across the entire time window or in selectable time periods. Frequency domain data can also be obtained using fast Fourier transforms (FFT) and selectable windowing functions to quantify emission spectra. The EchoMaster program provides comparisons of (1) two individual emissions, (2) the means of two groups of emissions with up to 60 emissions in each group, and (3) an individual emission with its estimated background noise. An example of the data obtained from the EchoMaster analysis is shown in Figure 3–2.

Prior to addition of data, like conditions (i.e., the three conditions without noise and the three conditions with noise) are reviewed for data

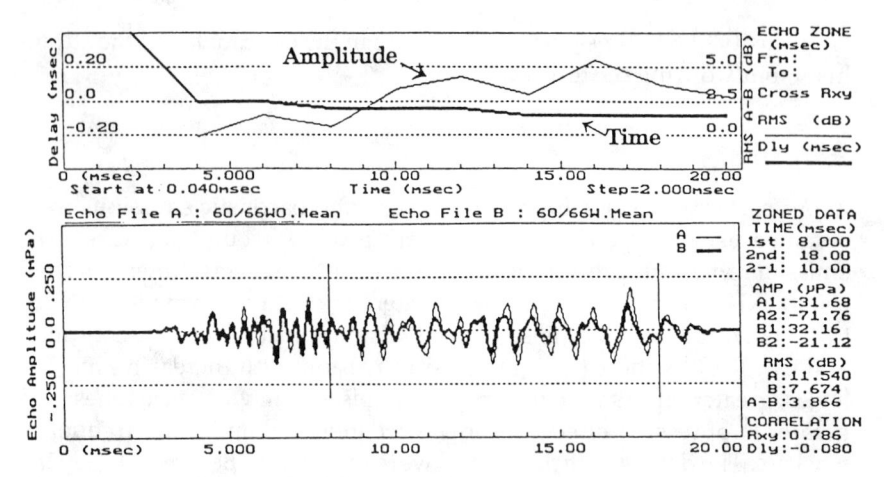

Figure 3–2. Analysis method for quantification of suppression using the Kresge EchoMaster program. Emissions obtained without (thin line) and with (thick line) are shown in the bottom portion. The top portion shows amplitude and time differences between the without and with conditions in 2-ms intervals.

consistency. Mean data are obtained for emissions from like conditions (i.e., without or with noise) only within subjects, and each subject's emissions are compared only with his or her own emissions. Once emission suppression is quantified for individual subjects through the EchoMaster analysis, we then can compare data across subjects.

CHARACTERISTICS OF TEOAE SUPPRESSION

What Are the Characteristics of Suppression in Normal Individuals?

Suppression of TEOAEs is characterized as a reduction in amplitude and/or a time change or phase shift (e.g., Berlin et al., 1993a; Collet et al., 1990; Ryan et al., 1991; Veuillet et al., 1991). Subjects vary in the amount of suppression, although in our experience all normal subjects show amplitude decreases with noise in some time periods. Some subjects demonstrate suppression of as much as 5 to 7 dB. As the intensity of the contralateral noise increases, the amount of suppression increases and time periods involved tend to broaden.

Suppression also is demonstrated as a change in the time of occurrence of peaks or zero crossings in the emissions, particularly at later time periods. Introduction of contralateral noise causes a decrease in the latency of peaks relative to the stimulus, or a "negative" time delay. This can be seen in the lower tracing of Figure 3–2 where the peaks in the suppressed condition are slightly earlier, particularly in later time periods. As the intensity of the contralateral noise increases, earlier time periods tend to be involved as well for both amplitude and time differences (Hood, Hurley, Wen, Berlin, & Jackson, 1993).

Test-retest reliability analyses have been incorporated into many of our studies of suppression. Results indicate good repeatability of suppression effects for both amplitude and time within subjects as well as consistent group effects (e.g., Hood et al., 1993).

Is Suppression Greater in Certain Time Periods?

A consistent observation throughout our studies is the occurrence of maximal suppression in the 8- to 18-ms time period which is consistent with other reports (e.g., Collet et al., 1990). Analysis by 2 ms intervals, as shown in Figure 3–3, indicates that suppression varies across time and that the greatest amplitude suppression and time delay changes occur in the time period between 8 and 18 ms. In this figure, data obtained from the EchoMaster analysis of a series of normal subjects have been combined to examine mean suppression effects on amplitude (left panel) and time (right panel). Very little suppression is observed from 2 to 8 ms in either the amplitude or time graphs. Effects across this group of subjects increase with time and are greatest in the 8- to 18-ms regions. Boxes outline the time window that is used to quantify suppression effects in our subsequent studies.

The "Echo in dB" value from the ILO88 system describes the characteristics of an entire emission as a single value. Because suppression effects are greater in some regions than in others, a single value cannot adequately represent the maximal effects or define time regions containing the greatest amount of suppression. In fact, an overall aggregate number will underestimate the suppression effect in most subjects. Thus, we recommend point-by-point analysis of suppression at 1-, 2-, or 3-ms time intervals to identify time regions of maximum effect and more precise quantification of suppression.

An example of a subject with minimal suppression when analyzed with the overall ILO88 number is shown in Figure 3–4. Although this single number might suggest the lack of a suppression effect, this subject shows substantial suppression between 10 and 12 ms. In addition, some subjects show greater amplitude changes while other subjects may show greater temporal changes.

Do Intensity Levels of the Click and Noise Affect Suppression?

We reasoned that because otoacoustic emissions are associated with cochlear processes occurring in response to low-intensity stimuli, it is

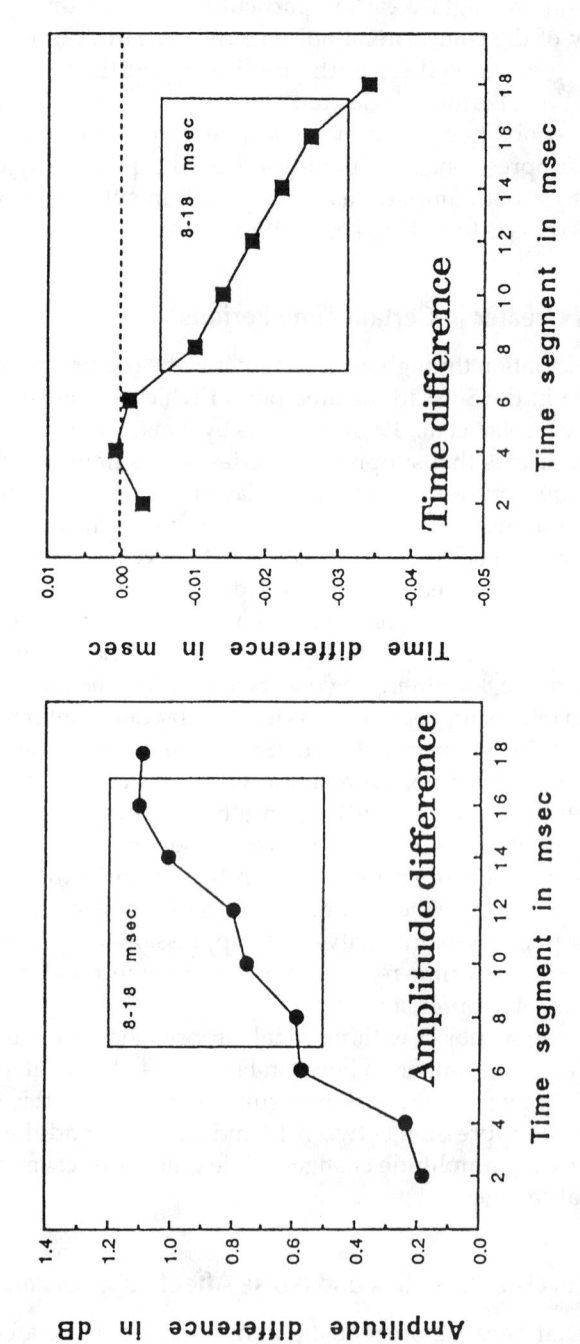

Figure 3–3. Mean data from a group of normal subjects show maximal amplitude (left) and time (right) differences in the 8- to 18-ms time window.

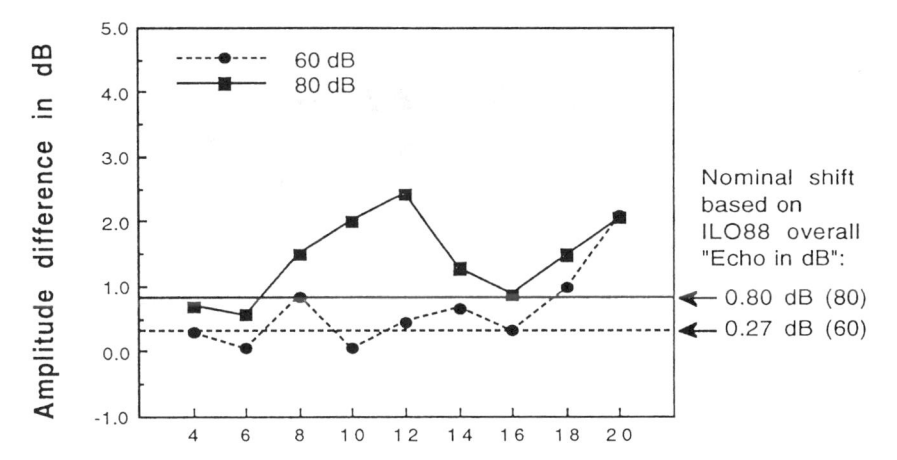

Figure 3–4. Some normal subjects who appear to have little contralateral suppression calculated in overall dB by the ILO88 system show clear amplitude changes in isolated time periods. Shown are data for one subject who shows less than 1 dB of suppression in the aggregate echo but more than 2.4 dB suppression in the 10–12 ms time period.

possible that fainter click and noise levels may be optimal for observing suppression effects. In one study, we varied the intensity of both linear clicks and contralaterally presented continuous white noise to determine the optimal click and noise levels that would yield the greatest contralateral suppression effect (Hood, Berlin, Hurley, Cecola, & Bell, 1994).

Comparison of suppression for linear clicks of peak sound pressures from 50 to 70 dB and contralateral white noise from 10 dB below to 10 dB above the click peak SP showed that the amount of suppression is dependent on both the level of the suppressor noise and the level of the stimulus eliciting the emission. Suppression increased systematically as the level of the noise was increased. Maximum suppression was reached with clicks of 55 dB peak SP and above (Figure 3–5). The observation of a decrease in suppression for 65 dB peak SP clicks suggests the possibility of different "low" and "high" level processes affecting suppression, depending on the stimulus and noise intensities.

The occurrence of greater suppression for some lower rather than higher intensity stimuli described here also reduces concern about contamination of suppression by either acoustic crosstalk or acoustic reflexes, both of which may contribute at high intensities but could not have a greater effect at lower than higher intensities.

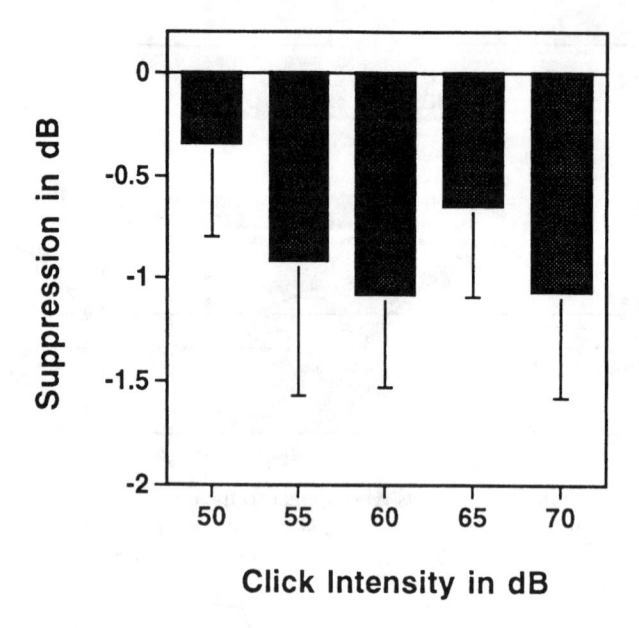

Figure 3–5. Effects of stimulus and suppressor intensity on suppression. The amount of suppression increases with increasing suppressor intensity, but is greater for some lower intensity stimuli.

BINAURAL, IPSILATERAL, AND CONTRALATERAL SUPPRESSION

The olivocochlear system can alter outer hair cell activity when activated by contralateral, ipsilateral, or bilateral stimuli. Although most experiments on suppression of otoacoustic emissions have involved contralateral simultaneous stimuli, Berlin, Hood, Hurley, Wen, and Kemp (1995) extended TEOAE suppression studies to the presentation of ipsilateral and bilateral suppressors as well as contralateral suppressors. In order to accomplish this, it was necessary to develop a forward masking paradigm which allowed temporal separation of the suppressor and the emission evoking click. This was accomplished through the assistance of Dr. David Kemp, who provided the software necessary to complete a forward masking paradigm using the Otodynamics ILO88 system.

Forward Masking Paradigm

In a forward masking paradigm, the masker precedes the test stimulus in time. By separating the masker and stimulus in time, acoustic interaction of the two signals is minimized. Even though a masker precedes the test stimulus, psychophysical studies have shown that a masking effect persists for a short time after the cessation of the masker.

To study the effects of binaural, ipsilateral, and contralateral noise on suppression we collected TEOAEs in a forward masking paradigm using linear clicks at 65 dB peak SP and a 65 dB SPL white noise masker that was 400 ms in duration (Figure 3–6). Time separations between the offset of the noise and the onset of the first click of a four-click series were varied from 1 to 200 ms. Because the ILO88 presents stimuli in groups of four, the three clicks following the initial stimulus were each separated by an additional 20 ms. Thus, only the first click in the series was masked according to these delay times, a limitation that we are currently correcting with another paradigm which allows presentation of a single stimulus following the masker.

Do Ipsilateral and Bilateral Noise Stimuli Yield Results Similar to Contralateral Noise?

Binaurally presented noise resulted in significantly greater suppression than ipsilateral or contralateral noise (Figure 3–7) and contralateral noise was the least effective suppressor (Berlin et al., 1995). Consistent with previous studies, the greatest suppression occurred between 8 and 18 ms following stimulus onset. Mean maximal suppression effects were on the order of 3.0 to 3.5 dB for binaural noise, 1.5 to 2.0 dB for ipsilateral noise, and 1.0 to 1.5 dB for contralateral noise.

Does the Time Separation Between the Noise Offset and the Click Affect Suppression?

The literature from behavioral studies of forward masking indicates that the effectiveness of a masker decreases as the time separation between

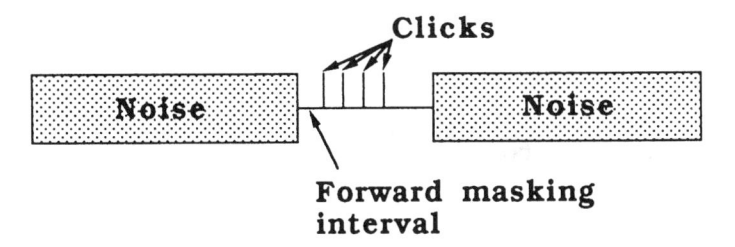

Figure 3–6. Diagram of a forward masking paradigm used to evaluate suppression of emissions.

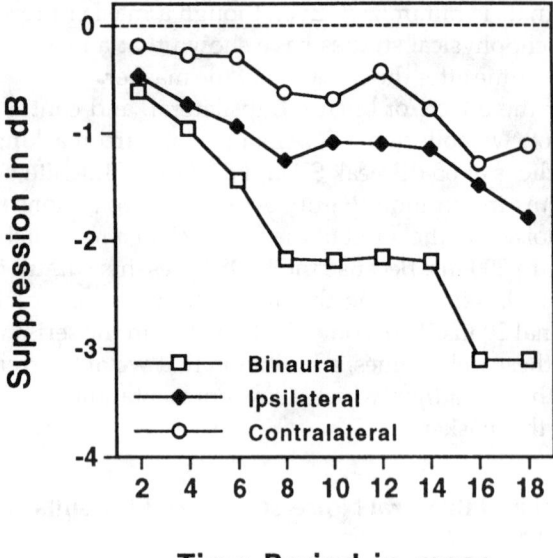

Figure 3–7. Comparison of suppression with ipsilateral, contralateral, and binaural noise. Binaural stimulation is more effective than either ipsilateral or contralateral noise.

the offset of the masker noise and the onset of the stimulus increases. Consistent with behavioral studies, the amount of emission suppression decreased systematically with increasing time separations between the masker and the click train (Berlin et al., 1995). One ms separation yielded the most suppression, and little or no suppression was observed when the noise and clicks were separated by 100 to 200 ms. It should be noted that these suppression effects may underestimate the actual suppression due to the additional time delay between the noise and the second, third, and fourth clicks in the train. When the time separation between a masker noise and a click is less than 10 ms, it is also possible that the noise itself will produce an emission that will contaminate the target response (Tavartkiladze et al., 1995). Thus, a time separation of 10 ms between the noise offset and stimulus onset appears to yield a suppression effect with minimized contamination.

Does Noise Duration Affect Suppression?

Liberman and Brown (1986) first showed that stimulation of 50 to 500 ms is required to obtain responses from olivocochlear neurons. For this reason, we investigated the effects of noise duration in a forward-masking paradigm on TEOAE suppression (Hood, Berlin, Wakefield, & Hurley, 1995). We compared broad-band noise durations from 80 to 640 ms (at 65 dB SPL) presented prior to the onset of 65 dB peak SP linear clicks. Increases in noise duration yielded progressively greater suppression through 400 ms with no significant increase in suppression for noise durations from 400 to 640 ms. These data extend to humans the observations made by Liberman and Brown (1986) that a minimum stimulus duration is necessary for activation of the efferent system.

Potential Problems and Other Considerations

Several factors have the potential to contribute to a reduction in emissions when noise is introduced. These include activation of the middle ear muscle reflexes and acoustic crosstalk or crossover of sound through the head. However, several factors reduce the possibility that either of these factors plays a major role in the observed suppression effects. Our data showing greater suppression effects for lower intensity stimuli minimize the potential role of the middle ear muscle reflex and crossover, as effects would be expected to increase with intensity if they represented either of these phenomena. Acoustic crossover is also unlikely because we used insert earphones with 60–90 dB interaural attenuation (Killion, Wilbur, & Gudmundsen, 1985). In addition, both our group and Collet and his colleagues have observed suppression in patients who lack stapedial muscle function due either to Bell's Palsy or stapedial tendon section during stapedectomy.

It is important to monitor click and noise levels during evaluation because these levels vary greatly across ears. Consistent with Collet and his colleagues, we also recommend use of linear rather than nonlinear clicks and presentation levels in the range of 55 to 60 dB peak SP in order to avoid the potential contaminants discussed.

Clinical Application

Based on our studies, we measure suppression of transient evoked otoacoustic emissions clinically using 55 or 60 dB peak SP linear clicks and noise levels of 55 to 65 dB SPL. We interleave three "without noise" and three "with noise" conditions, analyze results using the Kresge EchoMaster software, and focus on the 8- to 18-ms time period. In patients of interest, we present bilateral, ipslateral, and contralateral noise in a forward masking paradigm. We believe that suppression of otoacoustic emissions provides insight into function of the efferent system and the interactions between the afferent and efferent pathways which allow us to distinguish central from peripheral hearing losses and manage both types of hearing disorders more accurately (e.g., Berlin et al., 1993b; Williams, Brooke, & Prasher, 1994).

SUMMARY

The series of studies summarized in this chapter provide information about some of the characteristics of suppression of transient evoked otoacoustic emissions in adults with normal hearing. These characteristics of suppression can be summarized as follows:

1. Suppression is characterized by amplitude decreases as well as time shifts of emission peaks.
2. Suppression is greatest in the 8- to 18-ms time period.
3. Some normal subjects who appear to have little or no suppression when a single value is calculated to represent the entire 20.48 ms period show clear suppression in the 8- to 18-ms range.
4. As the intensity of the suppressor noise increases, suppression amplitude and time differences increase.
5. Suppression is greater for lower intensity stimuli than for higher intensity stimuli.
6. Suppression is greater for binaural noise than for ipsilateral or contralateral noise.
7. Suppression is greatest for time separations of less than 10 ms and for noise durations greater than 400 ms.
8. Test and retest comparisons show that suppression effects are repeatable.
9. Suppression of otoacoustic emissions is useful clinically in evaluating and managing patients with central and peripheral hearing losses.

Acknowledgment: This work was supported by NIH NIDCD P01-DC00379, DOD-DAMD1783V3013, Kam's Fund for Hearing Research, the Kleberg Foundation, and the Louisiana Lions Eye Foundation. We extend appreciation to David T. Kemp, Ph.D. for providing the forward masking software. We also acknowledge the following individuals for their participation in data collection: Betsey Bell, M.C.D., R. Patrick Cecola, M.D., Dena Jackson, M.A.T., Laura Wakefield, M.A.

REFERENCES

Berlin, C. I., Hood, L. J., Cecola, R. P., Jackson, D. F., & Szabo, P. (1993a). Does Type I afferent neuron dysfunction reveal itself through lack of efferent suppression? *Hearing Research, 65*, 40–50.

Berlin, C. I., Hood, L. J., Wen, H., Szabo, P., Cecola, R. P., Rigby, P., & Jackson, D. F. (1993b). Contralateral suppression of non-linear click-evoked otoacoustic emissions. *Hearing Research, 71*, 1–11.

Berlin, C. I., Hood, L. J., Hurley, A., Wen, H., & Kemp, D. (1995). Binaural noise suppresses linear click-evoked otoacoustic emissions more than ipsilateral or contralateral noise. *Hearing Research.*

Brownell, W. E., Bader, C. R., Bertrand, D., & de Ribaupierre, Y. (1985). Evoked mechanical responses of isolated cochlear outer hair cells. *Science, 227*, 194–196.

Buno, W., Jr. (1978). Auditory nerve fiber activity influenced by contralateral sound stimulation. *Experimental Neurology, 59*, 62–74.

Collet, L., Kemp, D. T., Veuillet, E., Duclaux, R., Moulin, A., & Morgon, A. (1990). Effect of contralateral auditory stimuli on active cochlear micro-mechanical properties in human subjects. *Hearing Research, 43*, 251–262.

Glattke, T. J., & Kujawa, S. G. (1991). Otoacoustic emissions. *American Journal of Audiology, 1*, 29–40.

Grose, J. H. (1983). The effect of contralateral suppression on spontaneous acoustic emissions. *Journal of the Acoustical Society of America, 74*, S38.

Hood, L. J., Berlin, C. I., Hurley, A., Cecola, R. P., & Bell, B. (1994). Intensity effects on contralateral suppression of linear click-evoked otoacoustic emissions. *Abstracts of the Seventeenth Midwinter Research Meeting, Association for Research in Otolaryngology, 17*, 52.

Hood, L. J., Berlin, C. I., Wakefield, L., & Hurley, A. (1995). Noise duration affects bilateral, ipsilateral and contralateral suppression of transient-evoked otoacoustic emissions in humans. *Abstracts of the Eighteenth Midwinter Research Meeting, Association for Research in Otolaryngology, 18*, 123.

Hood, L. J., Hurley, A., Wen, H., Berlin, C. I., & Jackson, D. F. (1993). A new view of contralateral suppression of transient evoked otoacoustic emissions. *Abstracts of the Sixteenth Midwinter Research Meeting, Association for Research in Otolaryngology, 16*, 102.

Kemp, D. T. (1978). Stimulated acoustic emissions from within the human auditory system. *Journal of the Acoustical Society of America, 64*, 1386–1391.

Kemp, D.T. & Chum, R. (1980). Properties of the generator of stimulated acoustic emissions. *Hearing Research, 2*, 213–232.

Killion, M. C., Wilbur, L. A., & Gudmundsen, G. I. (1985). Insert earphones for more interaural attenuation. *Hearing Instruments, 36*, 34–36.

Liberman, M. C. (1989). Rapid assessment of sound-evoked olivocochlear feedback: Suppression of compound action potentials by contralateral sound. *Hearing Research, 38*, 47–56.

Liberman, M. C., & Brown, M. C. (1986). Physiology and anatomy of single olivocochlear neurons in the cat. *Hearing Research, 24,* 17–36.

Martin, G. K., Probst, R., & Lonsbury-Martin, B. L. (1990). Otoacoustic emissions in human ears: Normative findings. *Ear and Hearing, 11,* 106–120.

Mott, J. B., Norton, S. J., Neely, S. T., & Warr, W. B. (1989). Changes in spontaneous otoacoustic emissions produced by acoustic stimulation of the contralateral ear. *Hearing Research, 38,* 229–242.

Mountain, D. C. (1980). Changes in endolymphatic potential and crossed olivocochlear bundle stimulation alter cochlear mechanics. *Science, 210,* 71–72.

Norton, S. J., & Widin, J. E. (1990). Evoked otoacoustic emissions in normal-hearing infants and children: Emerging data and issues. *Ear and Hearing, 11,* 121–127.

Probst, R., Lonsbury-Martin, B. L., & Martin, G. K. (1991). A review of otoacoustic emissions. *Journal of the Acoustical Society of America, 89,* 2027–2067.

Puel, J.-L., & Rebillard, G. (1990). Effect of contralateral sound stimulation on the distortion product 2F1-F2: Evidence that the medial efferent system is involved. *Journal of the Acoustical Society of America, 87,* 1630–1635.

Rabinowitz, W. M., & Widen, G. P. (1984). Interaction of spontaneous otoacoustic emissions and external sounds. *Journal of the Acoustical Society of America, 76,* 1713–1720.

Ryan, S., Kemp, D. T., & Hinchcliffe, R. (1991). The influence of contralateral acoustic stimulation on click-evoked otoacoustic emissions in humans. *British Journal of Audiology, 25,* 391–397.

Schloth, E., & Zwicker, E. (1983). Mechanical and acoustic influences on spontaneous otoacoustic emission. *Hearing Research, 11,* 285–293.

Tavartkiladze, G. A., Frolenkov, G. I., & Kruglov, A. V. (1995). Ipsilateral suppression of transient evoked otoacoustic emission (TEOAE). *Abstracts of the Eighteenth Midwinter Research Meeting, Association for Research in Otolaryngology, 18,* 122.

Veuillet, E., Collet, L., & Duclaux, R. (1991). Effect of contralateral acoustic stimulation on active cochlear micromechanical properties in human subjects: Dependence on stimulus variables. *Journal of Neurophysiology, 65,* 724–735.

Warr, W. B., & Guinan, J. J. (1978). Efferent innervation of the organ of Corti: Two different systems. *Brain Research, 173,* 152–155.

Warr, W. B., Guinan, J. J., & White, J. S. (1986). Organization of the efferent fibers: The lateral and medial olivocochlear systems. In R. A. Altschuler, R. P. Bobbin, & D. W. Hoffman (Eds.), *Neurobiology of hearing: The cochlea* (p. 333). New York: Raven Press.

Wen, H., Berlin, C. I., Hood, L. J., Jackson, D., & Hurley, A. (1993). A program for the quantification and analysis of transient evoked otoacoustic emissions. *Abstracts of the Sixteenth Midwinter Research Meeting, Association for Research in Otolaryngology, 16,* 102.

Williams, E. A., Brookes, G. B., & Prasher, D. K. (1994). Effects of olivocochlear bundle section on otoacoustic emissions in humans: Efferent effects in comparison with control subjects. *Acta Oto-laryngologica, 114,* 121–129.

4

Cochlear Outer Hair Cells vis-á-vis Semicircular Canal Type II Hair Cells

Charles H. Norris, Ph.D.
Tulane University School of Medicine
New Orleans, Louisiana

INTRODUCTION

This chapter briefly compares two types of hair cells from different organs of the inner ear. The purpose is to show their unique and very different characteristics and to suggest that these characteristics underlie the differing susceptibilities of these two cells to pharmacologic agents. It also suggests that we are on the threshold of a new era in otologic treatment wherein surgery and pharmacology have begun to combine their expertise to design new approaches to the old problems of tinnitus, various types of hearing losses, and vertigo.

Superficially the mechanoreceptors of the inner ear, the hair cells, all appear similar in structure and function (Figure 4–1). That is, bending of the cilia at the apical surface of the cells results in electrical changes within the cells and subsequent stimulation of the nerves making contact with these cells (Hudspeth, 1989). However, the methods of mechanical stimulation and final neural results are specialized within each inner ear endorgan. For example, in the membranous labyrinth (Figure 4–2), the semicircular canals respond to angular accelerations of the head, whereas the cochlea responds to sound pressures (Hudspeth, 1989). It is becoming apparent that these functional specializations may be largely controlled, or at least highly influenced, by the natural variations in the biophysical and biochemical properties of individual hair cells. In this regard, we have compared some of the properties of semicircular canal type II hair

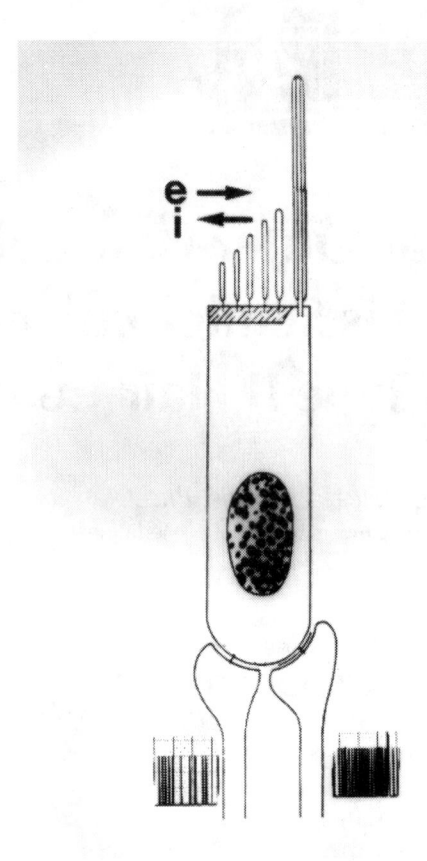

Figure 4–1. Cartoon of a universal inner ear hair cell. Pushing the cilia in one direction excites (**e**) and increases neural firing, whereas pushing in the opposite direction (**i**) reduces neural firing.

cells (SCC) to those of cochlear outer hair cells (OHC) (Ricci, Erostegui, Bobbin, & Norris, 1994). We have also noted their similarities and differences in susceptibility to the ototoxic effects of two members of the aminoglycoside family of antibiotics—streptomycin and gentamicin (Norris, Aubert, & Shea, 1994).

MORPHOLOGY

The sizes and shapes of the two types of cells are different (Ricci et al., 1994). OHCs are much larger than SCCs and appear uniformly cylindri-

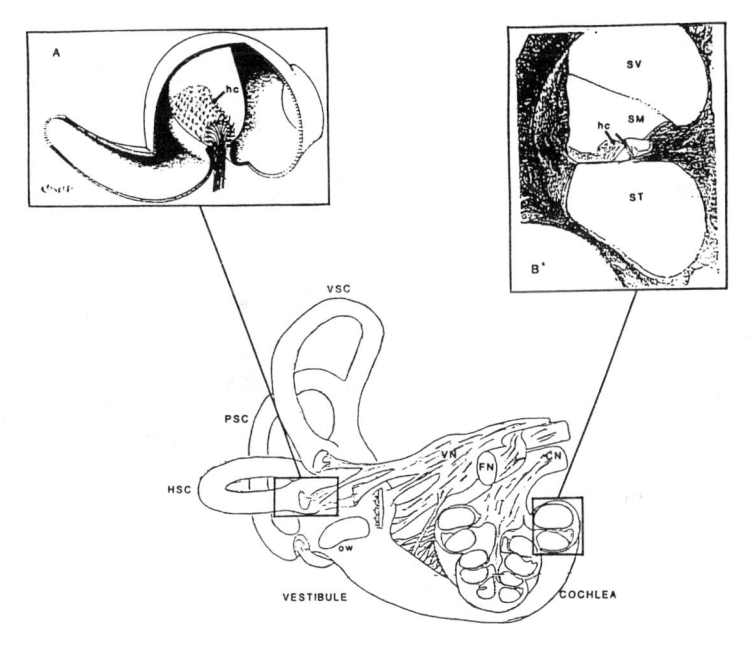

Figure 4–2. The membranous labyrinth with the cochlea dissected in a mid-modiolar plane. CN is the cochlear nerve, FN is the facial nerve, VN is the vestibular nerve, OW is the oval window, HSC is the horizontal semicircular canal, PSC is the posterior semicircular canal, VSC is the vertical semicircular canal, hc indicates hair cells, SV is scala vestibuli, SM is scala media, and ST is scala tympani. *Panel A* is an expanded view of the horizontal canal crista ampullaris and *panel B* is an expanded view of one turn of the cochlea.

cal in shape (Figure 4–3.). Only the lengths seem to vary when comparing one OHC to another. OHCs from the apical end of the cochlea are longer than those from the basal end, and OHC length also increases from the first outer row to the second and then third outer rows at a given place in the cochlea. In general, the shapes of OHCs that have not been stimulated look identical (Ricci et al., 1994). SCC shapes are more varied. They can be classified into at least three groups—cigar-, club-, and pear-shaped (Guth, Fermin, Pantoja, Edwards, & Norris, 1994; Figure 4–4).

In the frog, the cigar- and club-shaped SCC groups each make up about 40% of the total hair cells within a given crista ampullaris. The cigar- and club-shaped cells are found throughout the crista but are more numerous in the periphery, especially the cigar-shaped cells. The pear-shaped group accounts for about 20% of the total and are mostly all concentrated near the center of the crista. There is some minor overlap

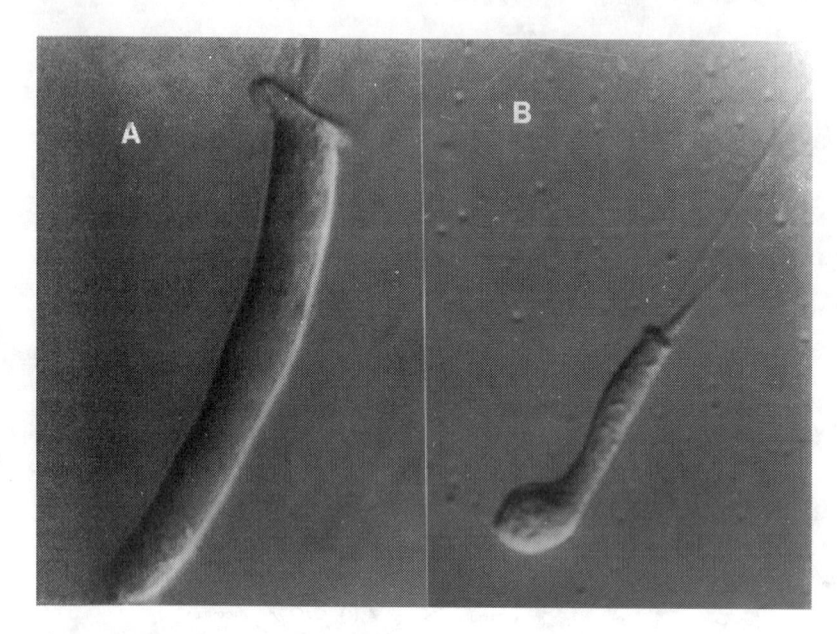

Figure 4–3. **A.** An isolated cochlear outer hair cell. **B.** An isolated semicircular canal haircell.

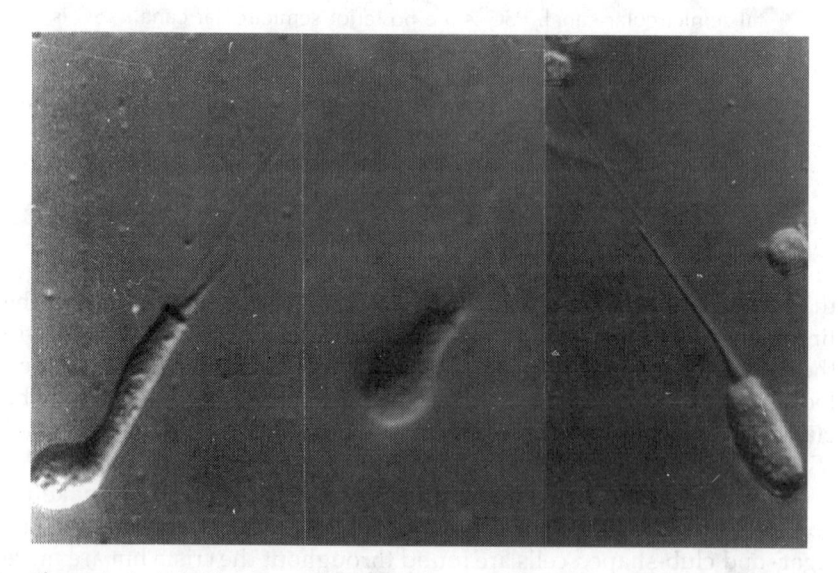

Figure 4–4. *Left:* Club-shaped semicircular canal hair cell. *Center:* Pear-shaped semicircular canal hair cell. *Right:* Cigar-shaped semicircular canal hair cell.

between these groups depending on the judgment of the observer. In addition to the previous structural differences, mature SCCs have a giant hair-like process called the kinocilium (Lowenstein, 1974), whereas mature OHCs are devoid of this structure (Nielson & Slepecky, 1986).

FUNCTION

The function of the OHCs is now thought to be related to a change of the stiffness properties in the basilar membrane in response to sound (Brownell, Bader, Bertrand, & de Ribaupierre, 1986; Kim, 1986; Ruggero, 1992). In the last 15 years it has become known that the mechanical properties of the basilar membrane in the cochlea are highly nonlinear and very sharply tuned. These mechanical basilar membrane properties can now account for almost all of the electrophysiologic responses of the auditory portion of the eighth nerve when the ear is stimulated by sound (Johnstone, Patuzzi, & Yates, 1986; Kim, 1986). There is rather strong support for the hypothesis that the enhanced and sharply tuned response of the basilar membrane is, in part, due to an active process in the outer hair cells (Johnstone, et al., 1986; Kim, 1986). The details are not yet clear as to how the active process is triggered or controlled or even in which part of the hair cell it resides. However, it seems safe to say that it is intimately linked to the transduction current and the subsequent cascade of events which follow mechanical movement of the stereocilia. This cascade includes opening and closing of ion channels in the walls of the outer hair cells, movement of free calcium, protein configuration changes, and release of neurotransmitters and neuromodulators. In isolated hair cell preparations, the outer hair cells can be made to change length and shape by a variety of stimulations (Brownell, et al., 1986; Cecola & Bobbin, 1992). Much research has been, and is currently, directed toward an understanding of how these mechanical changes in isolated hair cells may relate to the active process in the OHCs when they reside in the whole cochlear organ.

In contrast to OHCs, the SCCs provide the central nervous system (CNS) with neural signals that are proportional to the angular accelerations of the head (Lowenstein, 1974, Precht, 1978). When stimulated, SCCs do not appear to change length or shape. (However, the other mammalian semicircular canal hair cells, the type I hair cells, can do so [Didier, Decory, & Cazals,1990; Sans, Griguer, & Lehouelleur, 1994]).

Lowenstein and Sand (1940) were the first to demonstrate that the firing patterns in the nerves from SCCs in the Thornback Ray (*Raja clavata*) were directly proportional to angular accelerations of the head. Goldberg and Fernandez (1982) have reviewed the functions of the semicircular canals and describe the displacement of the endolymph and cupula as being proportional to angular accelerations at low frequencies of head movement (long durations of constant accelerations) and as being proportional to angular velocities at medium frequencies (short durations) of head movement. Most head movements are in the medium frequency range (Goldberg & Fernandez, 1982). As a general rule then, the neural responses from SCCs are related to these displacements of the endolymph and cupula.

ELECTRICAL PROPERTIES

OHCs have markedly different electrical properties as compared to SCCs (Ricci, et al., 1994; Table 4–1). OHC input resistance is about 95 MΩ whereas SCC input resistance is more than 3 times that—at about 400 MΩ. In accordance with their larger size OHC whole cell capacitance is approximately 36 pF as compared to the smaller SCCs which have around 10 pF of capacitance. In general, currents in OHCs are 3 to 7 times as large as those of SCCs but current density (currents normalized to surface area) is about the same for OHCs and SCCs being near 1.25nA/cm^2.

Both types of cells are dominated by potassium conductances in their cell walls. The aggregate K$^+$ conductance of the OHCs is almost linear over a wide range of membrane voltage and current, whereas the aggregate K$^+$ conductance of the majority of SCCs is inactivating (self-inhibiting) and outwardly rectifying (Ricci, et al., 1994; Figure 4–5).

Table 4–1. Summary of the various results obtained from the two cell types.

Characteristics	Outer Hair Cell	Semicircular Canal Hair Cell
Visible nucleus	Must be visible	Not visible
Opacity	Translucent	Opaque
Surface area	2244 ± 37 μM*	842 ± 18 μm
Input resistance	95 ± 11 MΩ*	386 ± MΩ
Whole-cell capacitance	36 ± 0.6 pF*	10.4 ± 0.7 pF
Specific capacitance	1.8 ± 0.2μF/cm^2	1.2 ± 0.4 pFcm^2
Zero-current potential	−44 ± 1 mV	−45 ± 1 mV
Peak current	2814 ± 100 pA*	1018 ± 75 pA
Peak current density	1.25 ± 0.03 nA/cm^2	1.2 ± 0.4 nA/cm^2
Late current	2630 ± 102 pA*	337 ± 25 pA
Late current density	1.17 ± 0.03 NA/cm^2	0.40 ± 0.01 nA/cm^2
Ratio (peak/late)	1.08 ± 0.01*	3.6 ± 0.3

*Significance at the P, 0.01 level using a two-tailed Student's t-test.

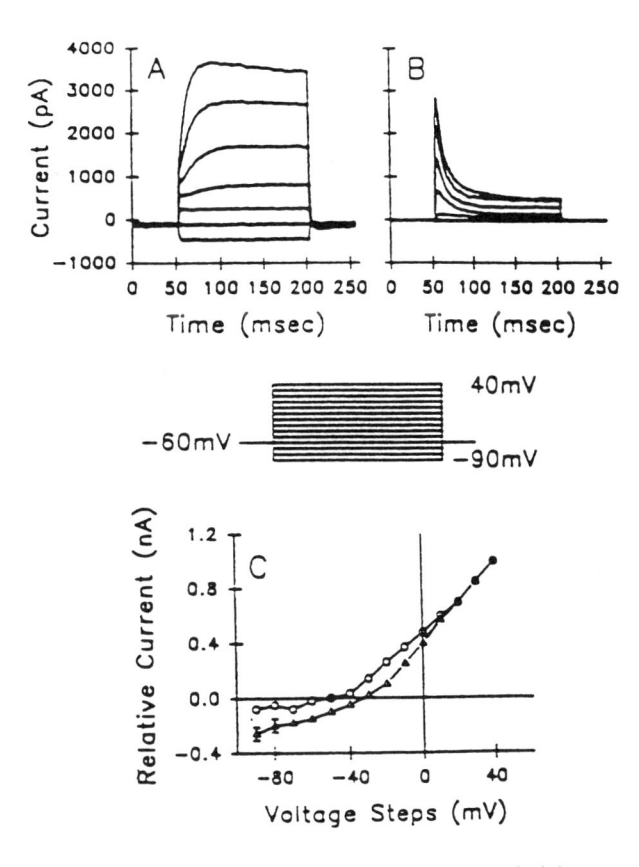

Figure 4–5. *Top:* Voltage-clamp currents recorded from a cochlear outer hair cell (A) and a semicircular canal hair cell (B). *Middle:* The voltage protocol used to elicit these currents. *Bottom:* Voltage-current plots based on the data shown at the top. Open circles are for the semicircular canal hair cell and open triangles are for the cochlear outer hair cell.

OHCs and SCCs have various Ca^{++}-dependent and Ca^{++}-independent K^+ conductances, outward rectifying K^+ conductances, L-type Ca^{++} conductances, inward rectifying K^+ conductances, and chloride conductances. However, the proportions, the single channel conductance value, the voltage sensitivity, and the activation and inactivation properties of each type of conductance are markedly different between the two types of cells (Housley & Ashmore, 1992; Housley, Norris, & Guth 1989; Ricci, et al., 1994).

INNERVATION AND RECEPTORS

Both OHCs and SCCs have efferent innervation which is primarily cholinergically mediated (Eybalin, 1993; Erostegui, Norris, & Bobbin, 1994; Norris, Housley, Williams, Guth, & Guth, 1988). The apparent response of the OHCs to efferent stimulation is a reduction in the associated afferent activity (OHC hyperpolarization; Figure 4–6) and the hair cell receptor is more nicotinic-like than muscarinic-like in its responses to various blocking agents (Erostegui et al., 1994).

In contrast, the response of SCCs to efferent stimulation is mainly excitatory (SCC depolarization) and is best blocked by atropine (muscarinic-like; Norris et al., 1988; Figure 4–7). When the SCC excitatory receptor is blocked, an inhibitory receptor is unmasked which has some

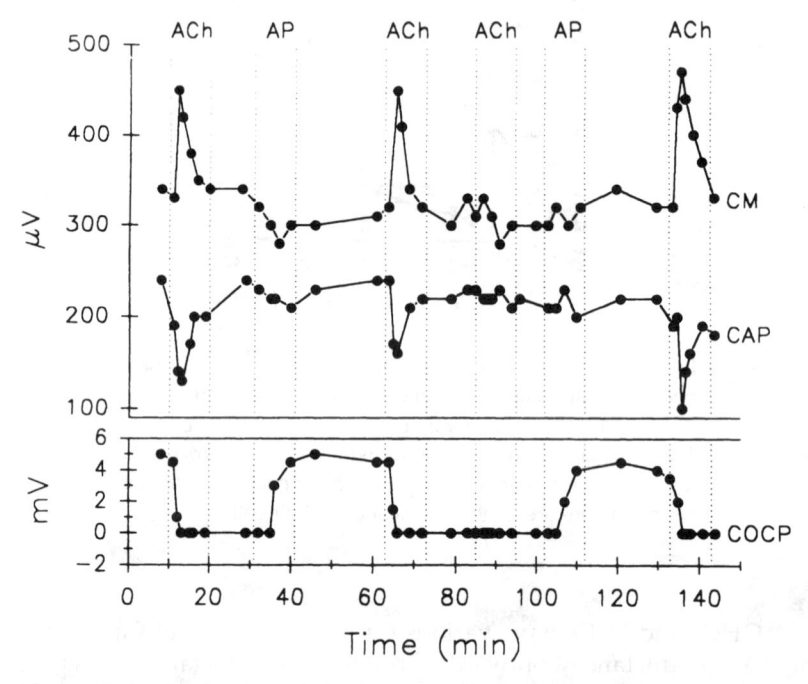

Figure 4–6. *Upper Panel:* Scala tympani perfusion of acetylcholine enhances cochlear microphonics but reduces the amplitude of the auditory nerve compound action potential (i.e., mimics efferent nerve stimulation). ACh = acetylcholine, AP = artificial perilymph, CM = cochlear microphonics, CAP = auditory nerve compound action potential. *Lower Panel:* Scala tympani perfusion of acetylcholine blocks the endocochlear potential response to electrical stimulation of the efferent cochlear nerves (COCP).

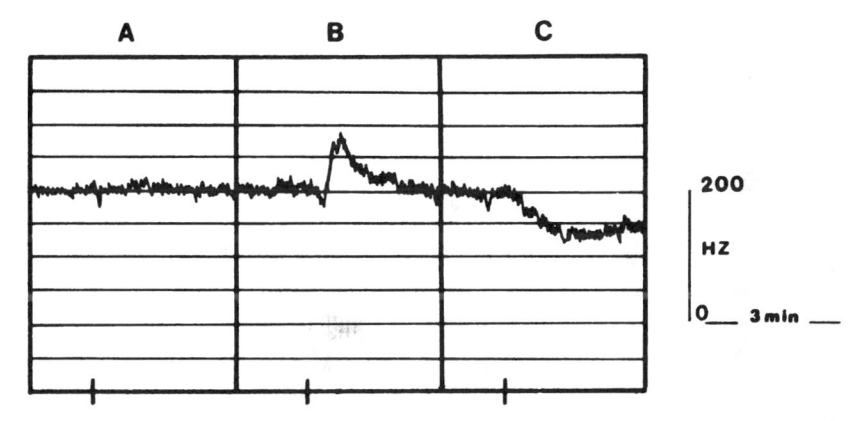

Figure 4–7. *Panel A:* Whole nerve spontaneous neural activity in a semicircular canal. *Panel B:* the increase in activity after injection of acetylcholine to the preparation. Between panel B and panel C atropine was added to the fluid bathing the preparation. *Panel C:* Injection of acetylcholine now causes a decrease in activity.

characteristics that are similar to the inhibitory receptor on OHCs (Norris et al., 1988). Morphologically, efferent innervation appears to predominate at outer hair cells in situ, whereas, in situ, SCCs appear to have a predominance of afferent innervation.

In addition to the efferent neurotransmitter receptors on these hair cells there are other neurotransmitter/neuromodulator receptors such as those for ATP, GABA, Glutamate, CGRP, Histamine, Enkephalins, dynorphins, adenosine, etc. (Eyebalin, 1993). These may not be important only for normal function of the cells but some may be vital for survival.

RESPONSES TO AMINOGLYCOSIDE ANTIBIOTICS

With all these differences between them, it is not surprising that SCCs and OHCs respond differently to various drug treatments. For example, although both types of cells can be acutely inhibited or destroyed by any individual aminoglycoside antibiotic, depending on the concentration and duration of the drugs in the inner ear fluids (Norris et al., 1993), SCCs are much more susceptible to streptomycin toxicity than are OHCs (Norris et al., 1993; Norris et al., 1994). Conversely gentamicin is relatively more toxic for OHCs than is streptomycin (Norris et al., 1994; Figure 4–8). The same relative toxicities obtain for both the long-term and the acute, reversible toxicities of these two drugs (Norris et al., 1994).

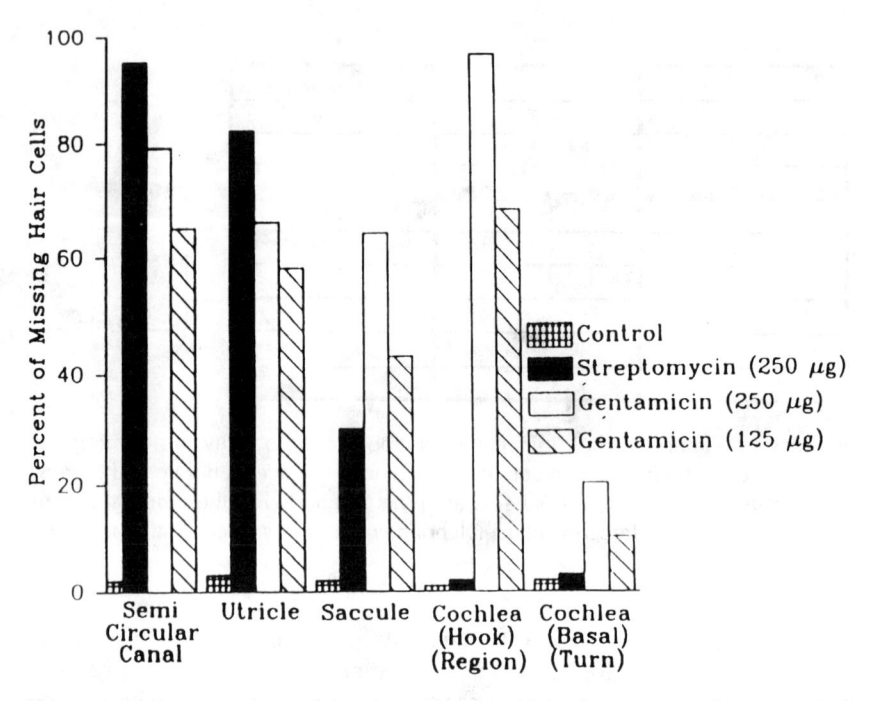

Figure 4–8. A comparison of the damage caused by gentamicin to that caused by streptomycin. Streptomycin is more toxic in the semicircular canals and utricle, whereas gentamicin is more toxic in the saccule and cochlea.

DISCUSSION

It is easy to speculate that one of the major advances in otologic treatment is going to be direct application of pharmacologic agents to the various organs within the inner ear. This has already begun in the case of ablation therapy (Beck & Schmidt, 1978; Norris, Amedee, Risey, & Shea, 1990). In some of these therapies drugs are being applied directly to the round window membrane (Beck & Schmidt, 1978; Figure 4–9) or to a fenestra in the lateral semicircular canal (Norris et al., 1990; Figure 4–10).

As seen previously there are important receptors, ion channels, and other structures on and within the hair cells and supporting cells that are vital to their function and that can be manipulated with pharmacological agents. With direct application of drugs to the cells, it will be possible to devise new therapies to abolish tinnitus, to resolve other abnormalities in hearing and vestibular function, and perhaps even to restore or replace dying hair cells. New surgical techniques and drug delivery systems are being rapidly developed for many medical problems and much of this

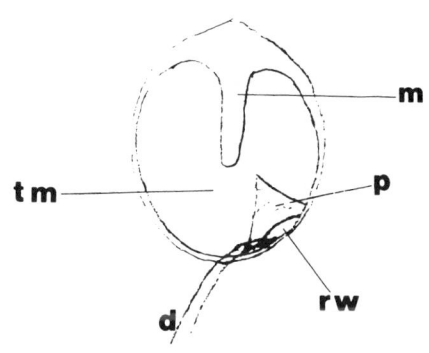

Figure 4-9. Application of a drug via a cannula placed in the round window membrane niche after making an incision in the inferior-posterior quadrant of the tympanic membrane. tm = tympanic membrane, rw = round window membrane, P = promontory bone over the basal turn of the cochlea, m = the manubrium of the malleus.

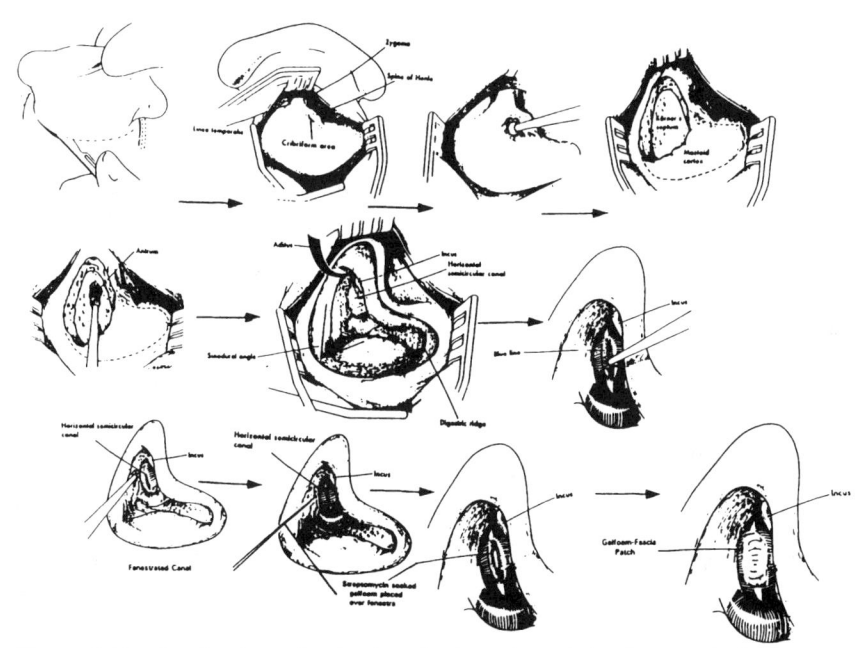

Figure 4-10. Application of a drug to the lateral semicircular canal after a post-auricular-mastoid approach has been made. *Top*: Posterior auricular incision exposing the mastoid bone. *Middle*: Drill-out exposing the horizontal and superior canals. *Bottom*: A fenestra is made in the horizontal semicircular canal and a drug-soaked piece of gelfoam is placed over the fenestra.

technology can be adapted for otology. Direct drug delivery and selectivity for particular otologic problems may be even more feasible when one considers that not only do hair cells from different inner ear organs have unique and significantly different properties, but hair cells from the same organ have differing properties (Norris, Ricci, Housley, & Guth, 1992; Steinacker & Romero, 1991).

Acknowledgments: This research supported in part by grants from The Research Institute for Hearing and Balance Disorders, Ltd., The Shea Clinic Foundation, and NIH NIDCD grants DC00722 and DC00303

REFERENCES

Beck, C., & Schmidt, C. L. (1978). 10 Years of experience with intratympanally applied streptomycin (gentamicin) in therapy of Morbus Meniere. *Archives of Otorhinolaryngology, 221*, 149–152.

Brownell, W. E., Bader, C. R., Bertrand, D., & de Ribaupierre, Y. (1986). Evoked mechanical responses of isolated cochlear outer hair cells. *Science, 227*, 83–90.

Cecola, R. P., & Bobbin, R. P. (1992). Lowering extracellular chloride concentration alters outer hair cell shape. *Hearing Research, 61*, 65–72.

Didier, A., Decory, L., & Cazals, Y. (1990). Evidence for potassium-induced motility in type I vestibular hair cells in the guinea pig. *Hearing Research, 46*, 171–176.

Erostegui, C., Norris, C. H., & Bobbin, R. P. (1994). In vitro pharmacological characterization of a cholinergic receptor on outer hair cells. *Hearing Research, 74*, 135–147.

Eybalin, M. (1993). Neurotransmitters and neuromodulators of the mammalian cochlea. *Physiological Reviews, 73*, 309–373.

Goldberg, J. M., & Fernandez, C. (1982). The vestibular system. In L. Darian-Smith (Ed.), *The handbook of physiology: Vol. 3. The nervous system: Part II. Sensory systems* (pp. 977–1022). Bethesda, MD: The American Physiological Society.

Guth, P. S., Fermin, C. D., Pantoja, M., Edwards, R., & Norris, C. H. (1994). Hair cells of different shapes and their placement along the frog crista ampullaris. *Hearing Research, 73*, 109–115.

Housley, G. D., & Ashmore, J. F. (1992). Ionic currents of outer hair cells isolated from the guinea pig cochlea. *Journal of Physiology, 448*, 73–98.

Housley, G. D., Norris, C. H., & Guth, P. S. (1989). Electrophysiological properties and morphology of hair cells isolated from the semicircular canal of the frog. *Hearing Research, 38*, 259–276.

Hudspeth, A. J. (1989). How the ear's works work, *Nature, 341*, 397–404.

Johnstone, B. M., Patuzzi, R., & Yates, G. K. (1986). Basilar membrane measurements and the traveling wave. *Hearing Research, 22*, 147–153.

Kim, D. O. (1986). Active and nonlinear cochlea biomechanics and the role of outer-hair cell subsystem in the mammalian auditory system. *Hearing Research, 22*, 105–114.

Lowenstein, O. E. (1974). Comparative morphology and physiology. In H. H. Kornhuber (Ed.), *Handbook of sensory physiology: Vol. VI/I. Vestibular system: Part I. Basic mechanisms* (pp. 76–120). Bethesda, MD: The American Physiological Society.

Lowenstein, O., & Sand, A. (1940). The mechanism of the semicircular canal. A study of the responses of single-fibre preparations to angular acceleration and rotation at constant speed. *Proceedings of the Royal Society B, 129*, 256–275.

Nielsen, D. W., & Slepecky N. (1986). Stereocilia. In R. A. Altschuler, R. P. Bobbin, & D. W. Hoffman (Eds.), *Neurobiology of hearing THE COCHLEA* (pp. 23–46). New York: Raven Press.

Norris, C. H., Amedee, R. G., Risey, J. A., & Shea, J. J. (1990). Selective chemical vestibulectomy. *American Journal of Otology, 11*, 395–400.

Norris, C. H., Aubert, A., & Amedee, R. G. (1993). The acute and chronic effects of streptomycin applied to the lateral semicircular canal. *American Journal of Otology, 14*, 373–377.

Norris, C. H., Aubert, A., & Shea, J. J. (1994). Comparison of cochleototoxicity and vestibulotoxicity of streptomycin and gentamycin. In M. Barbara & R. Filipo (Eds.), *Meniere's disease—Pathophysiology, diagnosis and treatment. Proceedings of the Third International Symposium, Rome, Italy 1993*. Amsterdam: Kugler Publications.

Norris, C. H., Housley, G.D., Williams, W.H., Guth, S. L., & Guth, P. S. (1988). The acetylcholine receptors of the semicircular canal in the frog. *Hearing Research, 32*, 197–206.

Norris, C. H., Ricci, A. J., Housley, G. D., & Guth, P. S. (1992). The inactivating potassium currents of hair cells isolated from the crista ampullaris of the frog. *Journal of Neurophysiology, 68*, 1642–1653.

Precht, W. (1978). Neuronal operations of the vestibular system. In H. B. Barlow, E. Florey, O. J. Grusser, & H. Van der Loos (Eds.), *Studies in brain function (Vol. 2*, pp. 3–48). New York: Springer-Verlag.

Ricci, A. J., Erostegui, C., Bobbin, R. P., & Norris, C. H. (1994). Comparative electrophysiological properties of guinea pig *(Cavia cobaya)* outer hair cells and frog *(Rana pipiens)* semicircular canal hair cells. *Comparative Biochemistry and Physiology, 107A*, 13–21.

Ruggero, M. (1992). Responses to sound of the basilar membrane of the mammalian cochlea. *Current Opinion in Neurobiology, 2*, 449–456.

Sans, A., Griguer, C., & Lehouelleur, J. (1994). The vestibular type I hair cells: A self regulated system? *Acta Otolaryngologica (Stockholm)*, (Suppl.) *513(Suppl).*, 11–14.

Steinacker, A. & Romero, A. (1991). Characterization of voltage-gated and calcium-activated potassium currents in toadfish saccular hair cells. *Brain Research, 556*, 22–32.

5

Genetics and Hair Cell Loss

Bronya J. B. Keats, Ph.D.
Nassim Nouri, M.S.
Jer-Min Huang, M.D.
Matthew Money, M.D.
Douglas B. Webster, Ph.D.
Mary Z. Pelias, Ph.D.
Charles I. Berlin, Ph.D.
Molecular and Human
Genetics Center
Kresge Hearing Research Laboratory of the South
Louisiana State University Medical Center
New Orleans, Louisiana

The etiology of profound sensorineural hearing impairment in children is genetic in the majority of cases. Even when an environmental cause is indicated, predisposing genes are likely to play a significant role (Duyk, Gastier, & Mueller, 1992). The hearing impairment may be part of a genetic syndrome or it may occur without other associated features. This chapter will review the work we have done toward identifying one of the genes for Usher syndrome and the *dn* gene that causes deafness with no associated anomalies in the mouse. Hair cell loss and degeneration of the organ of Corti characterize both of these recessively inherited forms of hearing impairment. The mode of inheritance for most cases of congenital nonsyndromic sensorineural hearing loss is also autosomal recessive, and family studies demonstrate that many different genes cause this clinical phenotype (Brownstein, Friedlander, Peritz, & Cohen, 1991). This genetic heterogeneity complicates the search for the defective genes. One promising approach is to study families from isolated populations. For example, Guilford, Ben Arab et al. (1994) and Guilford, Ayadi et al. (1994) mapped genes for deafness to chromosomes 11 and 13 in a Tunisian population, while Friedman et al. (1995) studied an isolated Indonesian population and showed that the defective gene is on chromosome 17.

A complementary approach is to identify genes that cause sensorineural hearing impairment in the mouse. Cordes and Barsh (1994) recently isolated the gene responsible for the mouse *kreisler* mutation which results in deafness and loss of vestibular function. A gene *(dn)* that causes deafness with no obvious associated anomalies was mapped to mouse chromosome 19 (Keats et al., 1995). The extensive homology between the mouse and human genomes means that such discoveries in the mouse provide insight into causes of hearing impairment in humans (Brown & Steel, 1994).

USHER SYNDROME

Several types of Usher syndrome have been distinguished by the severity and progression of clinical hearing impairment and vestibular dysfunction. Types I and II are the forms that are most widely recognized clinically (Möller et al., 1989). Usher syndrome type I is characterized by profound congenital hearing loss and vestibular dysfunction, Usher type II by moderate hearing loss and normal vestibular function (Smith et al., 1994). Cases of Usher syndrome in which the hearing loss is progressive have also been described and they are designated as Usher syndrome type III (Davenport & Omenn, 1977). All patients with Usher syndrome develop pigmentary retinopathy, but both the age of onset and rate of progression are variable. Histopathological studies of temporal bones of Usher patients show severe degeneration of the organ of Corti and spiral ganglion (Cremers & Dellerman, 1988; Shinkawa & Nadol, 1986).

Family studies of the three types of Usher syndrome have demonstrated genetic as well as clinical heterogeneity. Three genes for type I have been localized to chromosomes 11p (Smith et al., 1992), 11q (Kimberling et al., 1992), and 14q (Kaplan et al., 1992). Weil et al. (1995) showed that the 11q gene encodes the protein, myosin VIIA. Kimberling et al. (1990) and Lewis, Otterud, Stauffer, Lalouel, & Leppert (1990) assigned a gene for type II to chromosome 1q, and a gene for type III was localized to chromosome 3q (Sankila et al., 1995). Our studies have concentrated on the 11p locus for type I Usher syndrome in families of Acadian ancestry.

The Acadians

In the early 1600s French fishermen from the northern coastal regions of France (Brittany, Normandy) settled in the Canadian territory known as Acadia (now Nova Scotia and surrounding areas). According to Rushton

(1979), their population size grew from a few hundred up to nearly 20,000 by 1755 when the English ordered their expulsion from Acadia known as "Le Grand Dérangement des Acadiens." The Acadians were dispatched to Maryland, the Carolinas, and Georgia as well as to French ports and the West Indies; over the next 40 years about 4,000 Acadians made their way from these places to Louisiana. At first they settled along the banks of the Mississippi River above New Orleans, but with the Louisiana Purchase in 1803 and statehood in 1812 they were forced west across the Atchafalaya Basin, a 20-mile-wide, almost-impenetrable swamp. They settled on the plains among the bayous of southwestern Louisiana and remained relatively isolated because of linguistic, religious, and cultural cohesiveness, as well as geographic isolation. This population structure has resulted in higher frequencies of several recessive genetic diseases, including Usher syndrome type I, in the Acadian population than in the general population. We found 12 nuclear families in which at least two siblings had Usher syndrome type I and 15 families with one affected offspring. All of these 27 families were known to be of Acadian ancestry and they included a total of 46 affected individuals.

Linkage Analysis

Blood samples were drawn from affected individuals and their parents and unaffected siblings, and DNA was obtained by standard phenol-chloroform extraction methods. The DNA samples from all family members were genotyped for a set of 7 genetic markers known to be in the region of the Acadian Usher type I locus (USH1C) on the short arm of chromosome 11. These markers are designated as D11S569, D11S861, D11S419, D11S1397, D11S921, D11S1310, D11S899. The order of these markers is known from analyses of the Usher families as well as others (Keats, Nouri, Pelias, Deininger, & Litt, 1994). Genotyping was done using the polymerase chain reaction (PCR) followed by electrophoresis on a 5% denaturing polyacrylamide sequencing gel for about 2 hours. The PCR reaction mixture included 80 ng of DNA, 50 ng of each primer, one of which was end-labeled with ATP[γ-^{32}P], 200 μM dNTPs, and 1 U of *Taq* polymerase, together with magnesium chloride of optimal concentration (1.5–8.0 mM). The times and temperatures for 35 cycles of denaturing, annealing, and extension were 15 seconds at 94°C, 20 seconds at about 55°C, and 20 seconds at 72°C, respectively, with a final extension for 2 minutes at 72°C. DNA fragments (alleles) were visualized by overnight autoradiography.

Figure 5–1 shows an example of the results for the marker D11S921. Each of the affected offspring is homozygous for the 4 allele, while the two unaffected offspring have genotypes *4/5* and *5/6*. Similar results were found in all families, demonstrating that recombination did not occur between D11S921 and USH1C. The absence of recombination provides strong evidence that D11S921 is very close to the USH1C locus. Based on this result we can predict with high probability that the unaffected offspring who has the *4/5* genotype for D11S921 in Figure 5–1 is a carrier of the disease allele at the USH1C locus, while the unaffected offspring who has the *5/6* genotype for D11S921 has two normal alleles at the USH1C locus. Members of all of the families were genotyped for other markers in the region and Figure 5–2 shows a family in which recombination between D11S1397 and D11S921 is observed in one of the affected sons. The chromosomes that have the disease allele are shaded; the second affected offspring received part of the affected chromosome and part of the normal chromosome from his father. This result provides strong evidence that the USH1C locus is flanked on one side by the marker D11S1397.

In order to find a flanking marker on the other side of USH1C, we examined the alleles that were inherited with the disease alleles in each affected individual. Table 5–1 shows that the same D11S921 allele was

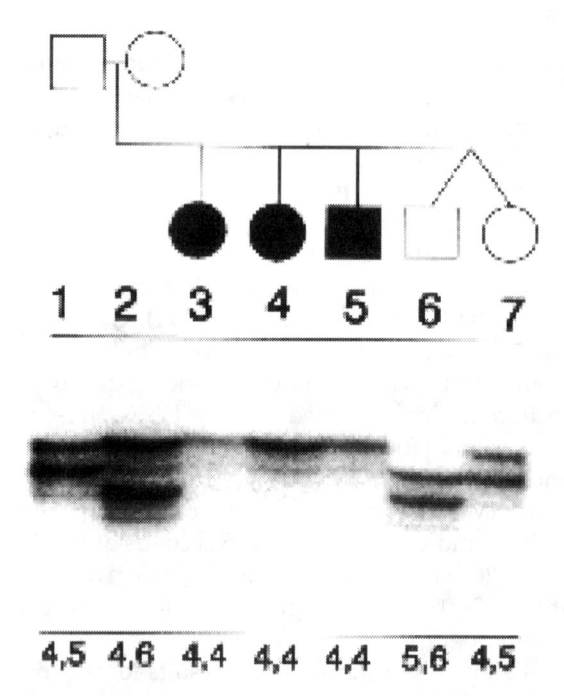

Figure 5–1. D11S921 genotype results for family in which three siblings have Usher syndrome type I.

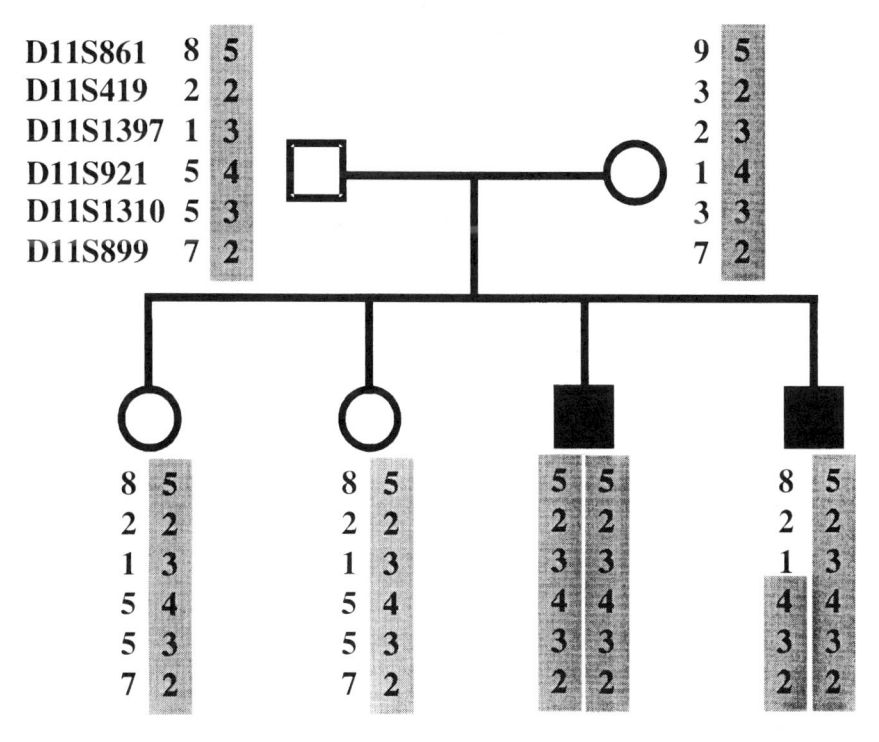

```
D11S861   8 5              9 5
D11S419   2 2              3 2
D11S1397  1 3              2 3
D11S921   5 4              1 4
D11S1310  5 3              3 3
D11S899   7 2              7 2
```

```
8 5    8 5    5 5    8 5
2 2    2 2    2 2    2 2
1 3    1 3    3 3    1 3
5 4    5 4    4 4    4 4
5 3    5 3    3 3    3 3
7 2    7 2    2 2    2 2
```

Figure 5–2. Family showing recombination between D11S1397 and D11S921 in an offspring with Usher syndrome type I.

TABLE 5–1. Marker alleles associated with the Acadian Usher chromosome.

D11S1397	D11S921	D11S1310	Usher	Non-Usher
3	4	3	49	4
1	4	3	1	0
3	4	4	2	1
1	4	4	1	1
3	4	5	1	0
Other			0	44
Total			54	50

found on all 54 chromosomes with the disease allele, but four of these chromosomes had a different allele at the D11S1310 locus. Thus, USH1C is likely to be between D11S1397 and D11S1310. Figure 5–3 shows the map giving the order of the markers and the distances between them measured in recombination units. A distance of one unit between two markers means that, on average, one recombination event is observed between these markers in a sample of 100 offspring. The region to which we have mapped this gene for Acadian Usher syndrome type I is about 1.2 recombination units which is probably less than 1.5 million base pairs of DNA, and we are continuing our efforts to isolate and characterize this disease gene.

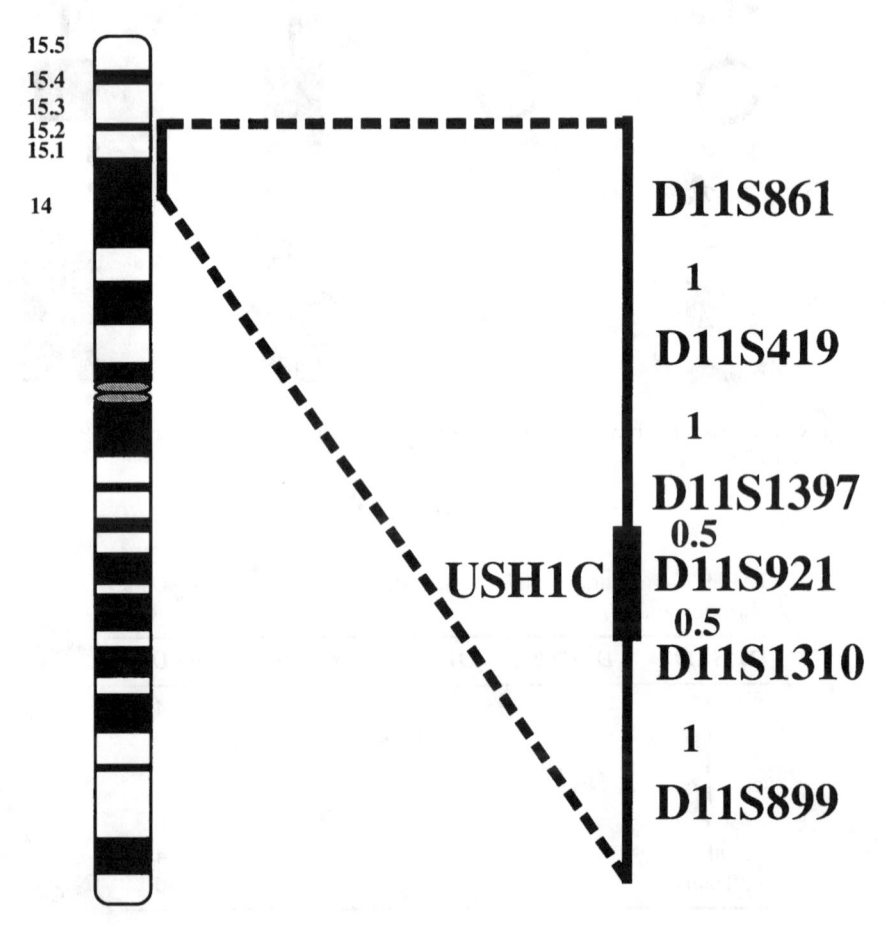

Figure 5–3. Map of chromosome 11 showing region that contains USH1C gene.

DEAFNESS (dn/dn) MOUSE

The *deafness* mouse has recessive sensorineural deafness with no other known physical or behavioral anomalies. This mutant was discovered in the curly-tail stock by Deol and Kocher (1958). They described early degeneration of the organ of Corti, stria vascularis, and occasionally the saccular macula. Pujol, Shnerson, Lenoir, and Deol (1983) showed that ultrastructural abnormalities of the inner hair cells are present at birth. By 15–20 days after birth the extracellular spaces of the organ of Corti are abnormal and there is significant loss of both inner and outer hair cells (Bock & Steel, 1983). By 45 days after birth the inner and outer hair cells have degenerated completely, and the organ of Corti has no distinguishable cell types from base to apex. However, Webster (1992) reported considerable regeneration of cells other than hair cells in the apical turn between 45 and 90 days after birth. Neither the mechanisms for degeneration nor regeneration are understood.

Matings

The localization of the gene *(dn)* causing deafness in the mouse requires a set of informative matings with affected offspring, and DNA markers, just as did the human studies to map the USH1C locus. In the mouse the task is simplified because large numbers of offspring can be obtained from any desired mating type. Matings were set up between male *deafness* mice and female *Mus musculus molossinus*. Both of these strains are inbred but the genetic divergence between them is high. Thus, the hybrid offspring are heterozygous for many markers making them highly informative for linkage studies. At the *dn* locus the *deafness* mice have the genotype *dn/dn*, while *Mus musculus molossinus* have two normal alleles, and the F_1 offspring must be heterozygous. These F_1 offspring were mated to *deafness* mice. Only two genotypes (each with 50% probability) at the *dn* locus are possible for each of the progeny from this mating; they must be heterozygotes if they can hear and homozygotes *(dn/dn)* if they are deaf.

Auditory Phenotyping

Fourteen matings between an F_1 hybrid and a *deafness* mouse were set up and 236 offspring were obtained. Each of these offspring was initially screened for a Preyer's reflex (ear "jump") in response to a sharp clap. If the mouse showed a reflex reaction it was classified tentatively as "hearing." The mouse was then anesthetized intraperitoneally and auditory brainstem responses (ABRs) were recorded from subcutaneous needle electrodes placed at the vertex and at the right retroauricular region, with the ground at the back. For each recording, 500 clicks were averaged with 1,000 times amplification and 100–3000 Hz filter bandpass. Screening for the Preyer's reflex categorized 120 of the mice as "hearing" and all of these mice had a normal ABR. We did not see a Preyer's reflex for the remaining 116 mice, and 113 of these mice had an absent ABR. However, 3 of them were reclassified as "hearing" based on a normal ABR. Thus, 123 were heterozygous at the *dn* locus and 113 were homozygous *(dn/dn)*.

Linkage Analysis

After the completion of the hearing tests the mouse was sacrificed and kidneys, spleen, and liver were obtained. DNA was isolated from homogenized kidney after standard proteinase K digestion and phenol-chloroform extraction, and the remaining organs were frozen. Each DNA sample was genotyped for DNA markers from the mouse genome following a protocol similar to that for the human markers. Genotypes were obtained for 230 samples. After genotyping these samples for 62 markers, we obtained strong evidence of linkage to the marker, *D19Mit14*, on chromosome 19. For all markers not on chromosome 19, approximately 50% of the offspring were recombinants. In contrast, no recombinants were found between the *dn* locus and *D19Mit14*. Other markers in the vicinity of *D19Mit14* were genotyped and the linkage map shown in Figure 5–4 was constructed from the data summarized in Table 5–2. These data provide the set of alleles on the chromosome inherited from the F_1 parent in each of the 230 offspring. The symbols M and D represent the alleles derived from the *M. m. molossinus* and *deafness* strains, respectively. Each F_1 parent must have the genotype M/D at all marker loci and each of the offspring inherited either the M allele or the D allele. Table 5–2 shows that no recombination was found with the markers *D19Mit14, D19Mit60*, and *D19Mit41*, while 7 recombinants were observed with *D19Mit28*, and 6 with *D19Mit96*, the closest flanking markers. The lack of recombination with 3 markers is consistent with the presence of an inversion on the chromosome carrying the *dn* gene. As in the case of the Acadian Usher syndrome type I gene, we are pursuing the isolation and characterization of the *dn* gene.

CONCLUSIONS

Etiological heterogeneity is found for many diseases including those that are known to be caused by a single gene mutation. Our studies demonstrate the value of isolated populations and mouse models for identifying genes that are responsible for diseases, particularly if the mode of inheritance is reces-

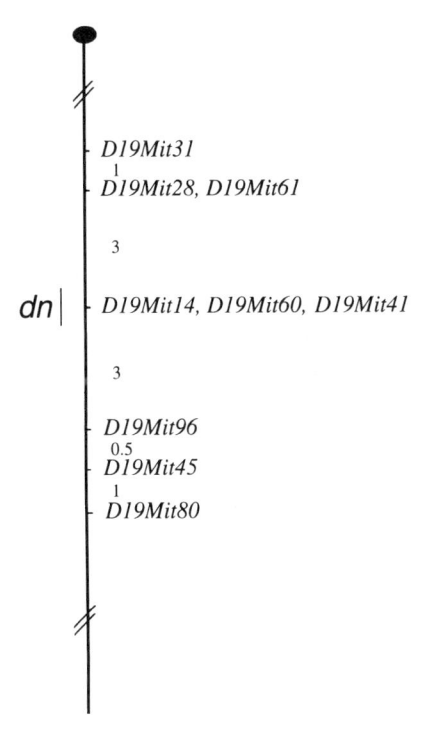

```
                    D19Mit31
                    │
                    D19Mit28, D19Mit61

                    3

   dn │             D19Mit14, D19Mit60, D19Mit41

                    3

                    D19Mit96
                    0.5
                    D19Mit45
                    1
                    D19Mit80
```

Figure 5-4. Map of mouse chromosome 19 showing region that contains *dn* gene.

TABLE 5-2. Alleles inherited from F₁ parent in 230 offspring. The symbols M and D represent the alleles derived from *M. m. molossinus* and *deafness* strains, respectively.

D19Mit31	D19Mit28/ D19Mit61	D19Mit41/ D19Mit14/ D19Mit60/dn	D19Mit96	D19Mit45	D19Mit80	Total
D	D	D	D	D	D	100
M	M	M	M	M	M	112
M	D	D	D	D	D	1
D	M	M	M	M	M	0
M	M	D	D	D	D	2
D	D	M	M	M	M	5
M	M	M	D	D	D	2
D	D	D	M	M	M	4
M	M	M	M	D	D	1
D	D	D	D	M	M	0
M	M	M	M	M	D	0
D	D	D	D	D	M	3

sive. The major advantage is that etiological heterogeneity is minimized, thus significantly increasing the chance of locating the defective gene.

Genes are responsible for the majority of cases of severe hearing impairment, and a genetic etiology needs to be considered for every patient with a hearing problem. Identification of genes for hearing impairment will provide alternative and complementary approaches to patient management. These genetic approaches will be important for prenatal testing, carrier detection, newborn screening, presymptomatic testing, and gene therapy. Most importantly our research will help to identify the basic genetic defects that cause hearing impairment.

GLOSSARY

Allele. One of the alternative forms of a gene or marker that is present at a locus. Different sized DNA fragments at a marker locus indicate the presence of different alleles.

Genotype. The pair of alleles present at a gene or marker locus in an individual.

Linkage. Loci on the same chromosome show linkage if the alleles are not transmitted independently from parent to offspring.

PCR. The Polymerase Chain Reaction (PCR) is a technique by which a short fragment (usually 100–300 base pairs) of DNA is amplified to make more than a million copies. The fragment to be amplified is specified by using flanking primers that are about 20 base pairs in length. An enzyme called a polymerase that is heat stable synthesizes new DNA strands. The reaction is repeated 30–40 times and with each cycle the amount of the DNA fragment of interest is doubled. Thus, large amounts of a particular DNA fragment can be obtained from a few nanograms of DNA.

Recombination. The observed alleles at a set of loci on an offspring's chromosome may be different from those observed on the parent's chromosome. This observation is probably recombination. Two loci show linkage if the frequency of recombination between them is less than 50%.

Acknowledgments: This work was supported by the Retinitis Pigmentosa Foundation Fighting Blindness, the Kleberg Foundation, and U.S. Public Health Service Grants DC00379 and DC00007.

REFERENCES

Bock, G. R., & Steel, K. P. (1983). Inner ear pathology in the deafness mutant mouse. *Acta Otolaryngologica, 96*, 39–47.

Brown, S. D. M., & Steel, K. P. (1994). Genetic deafness—progress with mouse models. *Human Molecular Genetics, 3,* 1453–1456.

Brownstein, Z., Friedlander, Y., Peritz, E., & Cohen, T. (1994). Estimated number of loci for autosomal recessive severe nerve deafness within the Israeli Jewish population, with implications for genetic counseling. *American Journal of Medical Genetics, 41,* 306–312.

Cordes, S. P., & Barsh, G. S. (1994). Positional cloning of *kreisler,* a mutation that causes deafness and segmentation abnormalities in mice. *American Journal of Human Genetics, 55,* A46.

Cremers, C. W. R. J., & Dellerman, W. J. W. (1988). Usher's syndrome temporal bone pathology. *International Journal of Pediatric Otorhinolaryngology, 16,* 23–30.

Davenport, S. L. H., & Omenn, G. S. (1977). *The heterogeneity of Usher syndrome* (Publication 426, abstract 215, pp. 87–88) Amsterdam: Excerpta Medica Foundation, International Congress Series.

Deol, M. S., & Kocher, W. (1958). A new gene for deafness in the mouse. *Heredity, 12,* 463–466.

Duyk, G., Gastier, J. M., & Mueller, R. F. (1992). Traces of her workings. *Nature Genetics, 2,* 5–8.

Friedman, T. B., Liang, Y., Weber, J. L., Hinnant, J. T., Barber, T. D., Winata, S., Nyoman Arhya, I., & Asher, J. H. (1995). A gene for congenital, recessive deafness DFNB3 maps to the pericentromeric region of chromosome 17. *Nature Genetics, 9,* 86–91.

Guilford, P., Ayadi, H., Blanchard, S., Chaib, H., Le Paslier, D., Weissenbach, J., Drira, M., & Petit, C. (1994). A human gene responsible for neurosensory, non-syndromic recessive deafness is a candidate homologue of the mouse sh-1 gene. *Human Molecular Genetics, 3,* 989–993.

Guilford, P., Ben Arab, S., Blanchard, S., Levilliers, J., Weissenbach, J., Belkahia, A., & Petit, C. (1994). A nonsyndromic form of neurosensory, recessive deafness maps to the pericentromeric region of chromosome 13q. *Nature Genetics, 6,* 24–28.

Kaplan, J., Gerber, S., Bonneau, D., Rozet, J., Delrieu, O., Briard, M., Dollfus, H., Ghazi, I., Dufier, J., Frezal, J., & Munnich, A. (1992). A gene for Usher syndrome type I (USH1) maps to chromosome 14q. *Genomics, 14,* 979–988.

Keats, B. J. B., Nouri, N., Huang, J. M., Money, M., Webster, D. B., & Berlin, C. I. (1995). The deafness locus *(dn)* maps to mouse chromosome 19. *Mammalian Genome, 6,* 8–10.

Keats, B. J. B., Nouri, N., Pelias, M. Z., Deininger, P. L., & Litt, M. (1994). Tightly linked flanking microsatellite markers for the Usher syndrome type I locus on the short arm of chromosome 11. *American Journal of Human Genetics, 54,* 681–686.

Kimberling, W. J., Möller, C. G., Davenport, S., Priluck, I. A., Beighton, P. H., Greenberg, J., Reardon, W., Weston, M. D., Kenyon, J. B., Grunkmeyer, J. A., Pieke Dahl, S., Overbeck, L. D., Blackwood, D. J., Brower, A. M., Hoover, D. M., Rowland, P., & Smith, R. J. H. (1992). Linkage of Usher syndrome type I gene (USH1B) to the long arm of chromosome 11. *Genomics, 14,* 988–994.

Kimberling, W. J., Weston, M. D., Möller, C. G., Davenport, S. L. H., Shugart, Y. Y., Priluck, I. A., Martini, A., & Smith, R. J. H. (1990). Localization of Usher syndrome type II to chromosome 1q. *Genomics, 7*, 245–249.

Lewis, R. A., Otterud, B., Stauffer, D., Lalouel, J. M., & Leppert, M. (1990). Mapping recessive ophthalmic diseases: Linkage of the locus for Usher syndrome type II to a DNA marker on chromosome 1q. *Genomics, 7*, 250–256.

Möller, C. G., Kimberling, W. J., Davenport, S. L. H., Priluck, I., White, V., Biscone-Halterman, K., Ödkvist, L. M., Brookhouser, P. E., Lund, G., & Grissom, T. J. (1989). Usher syndrome: an otoneurologic study. *Laryngoscope, 99*, 73–79.

Pujol, R., Shnerson, A., Lenoir, M., & Deol, M. S. (1983). Early degeneration of sensory and ganglion cells in the inner ear of mice with uncomplicated genetic deafness *(dn)*: Preliminary observations. *Hearing Research, 12*, 57–63.

Rushton, W. F. (1979). *The Cajuns: From Acadia to Louisiana*. New York: Farrar Straus Giroux.

Sankila, E. M., Pakarinen, L., Kääriäinen, H., Aittomäki, K., Karjalainen, S., Sistonen, P., & De la Chapelle, A. (1995). Assignment of an Usher syndrome type III (USH3) gene to chromosome 3q. *Human Molecular Genetics, 4*, 93–98.

Shinkawa, H., & Nadol, J. B. (1986). Histopathology of the inner ear in Usher's syndrome as observed by light and electron microscopy. *Annals of Otology, Rhinology, Laryngology, 95*, 313–318.

Smith, R. J. H., Berlin, C. I., Hejtmancik, J. F., Keats, B. J. B., Kimberling, W. J., Lewis, R. A., Möller, C. G., Pelias, M. Z., & Tranebjærg, L. (1994). Clinical diagnosis of the Usher syndromes. *American Journal of Medical Genetics, 50*, 32–38.

Smith, R. J. H., Lee, E. C., Kimberling, W. J., Daiger, S. P., Pelias, M. Z., Keats, B. J. B., Jay, M., Bird, A., Reardon, W., Guest, M., Ayyagari, R., & Hejtmancik, J. F. (1992). Localization of two genes for Usher syndrome type 1 to chromosome 11. *Genomics, 14*, 995–1002.

Webster, D. B. (1992). Degeneration followed by partial regeneration of the organ of Corti in deafness *(dn/dn)* mice. *Experimental Neurology, 115*, 27–31.

Weil, D., Blanchard, S., Kaplan, J., Guilford, P., Gibson, F., Walsh, J., Mburu, P., Varela, A., Levilliers, J., Weston, M. D., Kelley, P. M., Kimberling, W. J., Wagenaar, M., Levi-Acobas, F., Larget-Piet, D., Munnich, A., Steel, K. P., Brown, S. D. M., & Petit, C. (1995). Defective myosin VIIA gene responsible for Usher syndrome type 1B. *Nature, 374*, 60–61.

6

Hearing Aids: Only for Hearing-Impaired Patients with Abnormal Otoacoustic Emissions

Charles I. Berlin, Ph.D.
Linda J. Hood, Ph.D.
Annette Hurley, M.S.
Han Wen, M.S.B.M.E.
Kresge Hearing Research Laboratory of the South
Department of Otolaryngology and Biocommunication,
Louisiana State University Medical Center
New Orleans, Louisiana

The purpose of this chapter is to show that many patients have carried a misdiagnosis of "nerve damage" for years, a diagnosis that has semantically discouraged them from using hearing aids successfully. In fact, we can now discriminate between hair cell loss and primary neural disease and can consider using specialized types of dynamic compression hearing aids for patients with confirmed and isolated outer hair cell dysfunction. In contrast, patients with primary auditory neuropathies are *not* hearing aid candidates.

HOW DOES ONE DISCRIMINATE BETWEEN HAIR CELL AND NEURAL HEARING LOSS?

Outer Hair Cell Loss

Patients who have outer hair cell loss have audiograms that fall between 20 and 75 dB. Their otoacoustic emissions are absent, yet they have robust and synchronous neural discharges to clicks (Figure 6–1). This latter find-

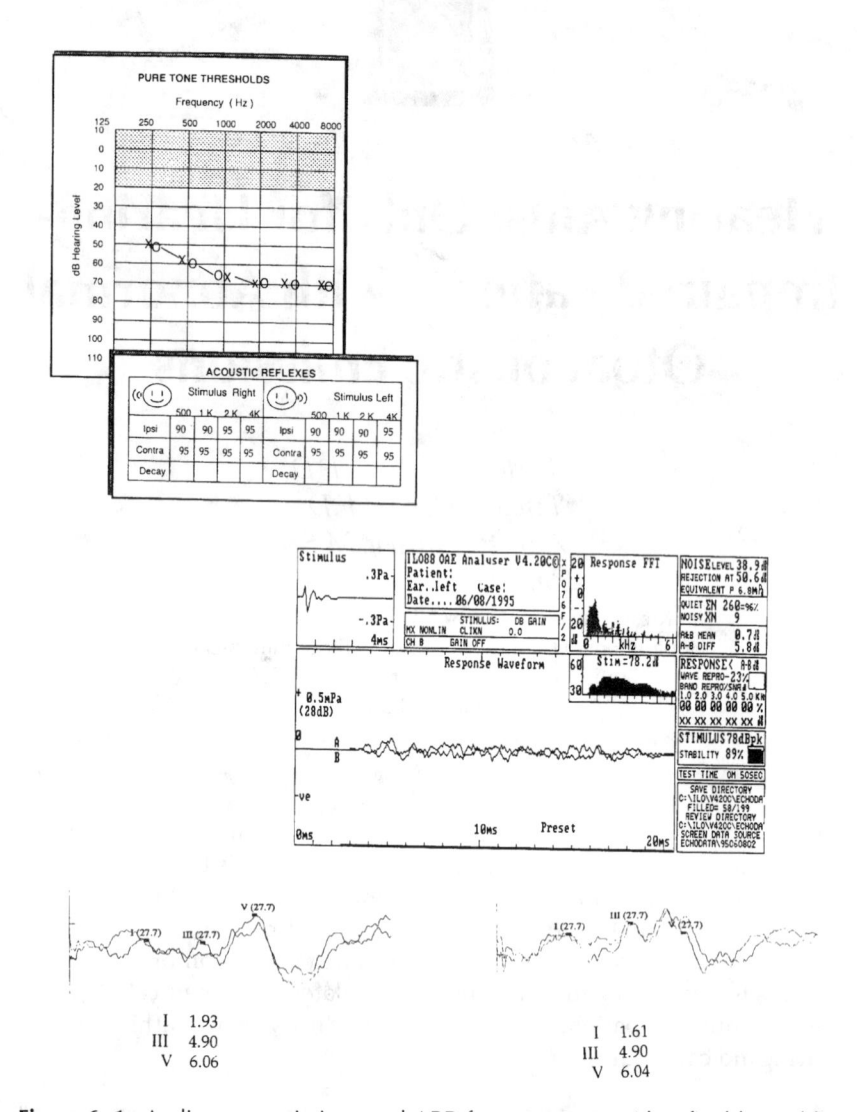

Figure 6–1. Audiogram emissions and ABR from a person with a fittable cochlear hearing loss.

ing is indicated by well-formed ABR responses with good morphology and normal absolute and interpeak latencies to high intensity, 85- to 95 dB HLn, stimuli. These are good candidates for hearing aids, and are likely to have good results, providing there are no inflammatory or autoimmune processes which disrupt speech coding.

Inner Hair Cell and Spiral Ganglion Loss

Patients who have no emissions and no ABR to air-conducted clicks are likely to have suffered some inner hair cell and spiral ganglion loss. If they are being considered for cochlear implants, electric ABRs should reveal synchronous neural discharge if properly administered and interpreted, thus, with somewhat circular reasoning, confirming their candidacy for cochlear implantation. However, many patients are successful implant candidates despite poor electrical ABR tests.

Primary Neuropathies

Finally, there is a small group of patients who have no ABR but have normal hair cell emissions. Some of these patients show little or no hearing loss by pure tone audiometry (Figure 6–2), others show very poor audiograms (Figure 6–3), still others have thresholds that fall somewhere in between (Figure 6–4). All show: (a) absent middle ear muscle reflexes, (b) absent MLDs, (c) very large otoacoustic emissions, and (d) virtually no efferent effects of contralateral ipsilateral or binaural noise on their robust click-evoked otoacoustic emissions (see sample in Figure 6–5 and explanation later; Berlin et al. 1994; Sininger, Hood, Starr, Berlin & Picton, 1995; Starr et al., 1991). Hood, Berlin, Hurley, and Wen have shown how we quantify efferent suppression in Chapter 3.

These patients probably have some form of primary auditory neuropathy which makes them poor candidates for hearing aids (Berlin et al., 1993, 1994) . Related evidence suggests that these patients also have other forms of nonauditory primary neuropathy like Charcot-Marie-Tooth syndrome or some similar disease that desynchronizes single unit responses in other motor as well as sensory units (Berlin et al., 1994; Sininger et al., 1995).

SUPPRESSION OF OTOACOUSTIC EMISSIONS

The medial olivocochlear system suppresses segments of outer hair cell activity when activated either contralaterally, ipsilaterally, or bilaterally with an auditory stimulus of sufficient duration (Kujawa et al., 1991; Liberman, 1989; Puel & Rebillard, 1990; Warr & Guinan, 1978; Warr, Guinan, & White, 1986).

In the previous chapter, Hood outlined our techniques for recording otoacoustic emissions and quantifying the efferent suppression that is the hallmark of the integrity of the afferent-efferent loop. In normal hearing subjects the suppression can approach 3 to 4 dB K, the designation we use

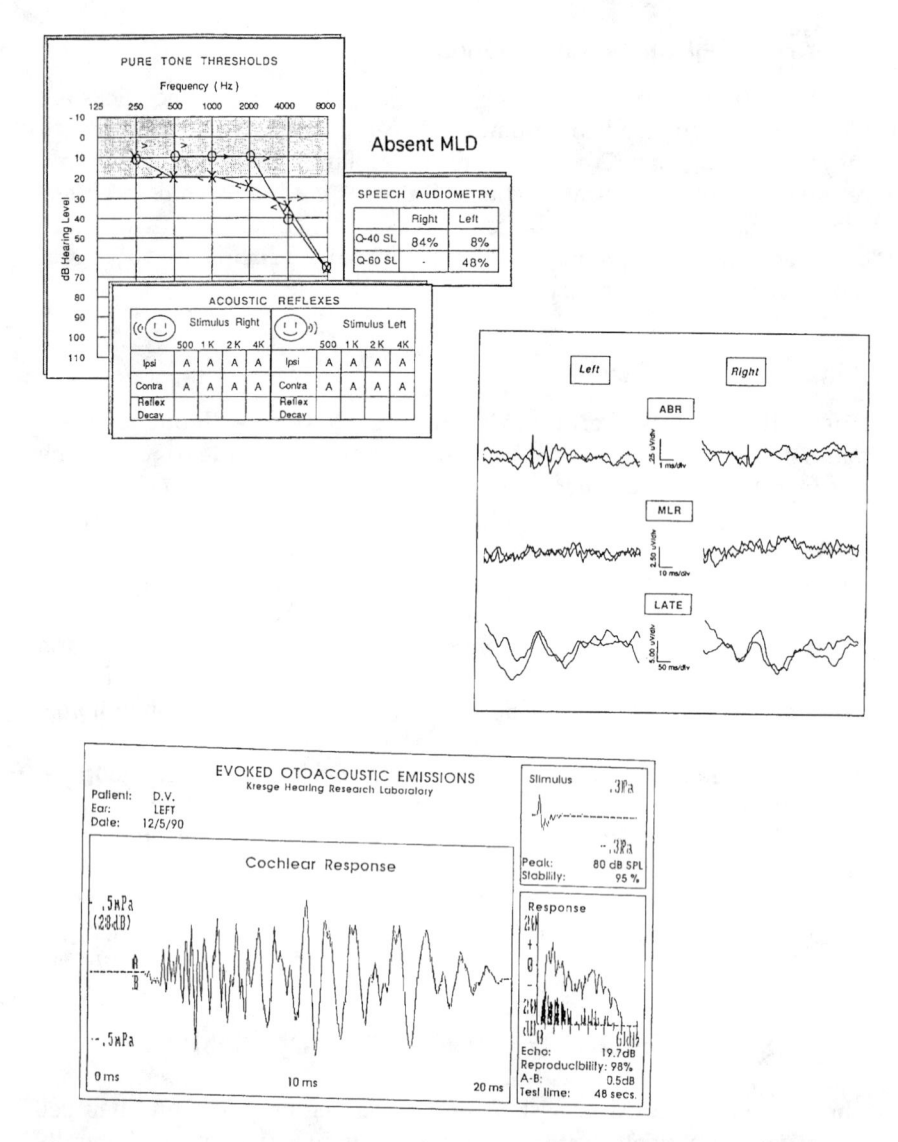

Figures 6–2 to 6–4. Audiograms and reflex are typical of those found in some patients with auditory neuropathy. Patients all have normal otoacoustic emissions and absent ABRs, MLDs, middle ear muscle reflexes, and poor speech discrimination in quiet as well as in noise. The patients universally showed no contralateral suppression when assessed by the Wen Kresge Echomaster Program. The kernel point is that the pure tone audiogram alone *cannot* be used to predict hearing aid need, success, or use, unless it is combined at least once with an otoacoustic emissions test showing absent or reduced emissions. *(continued)*

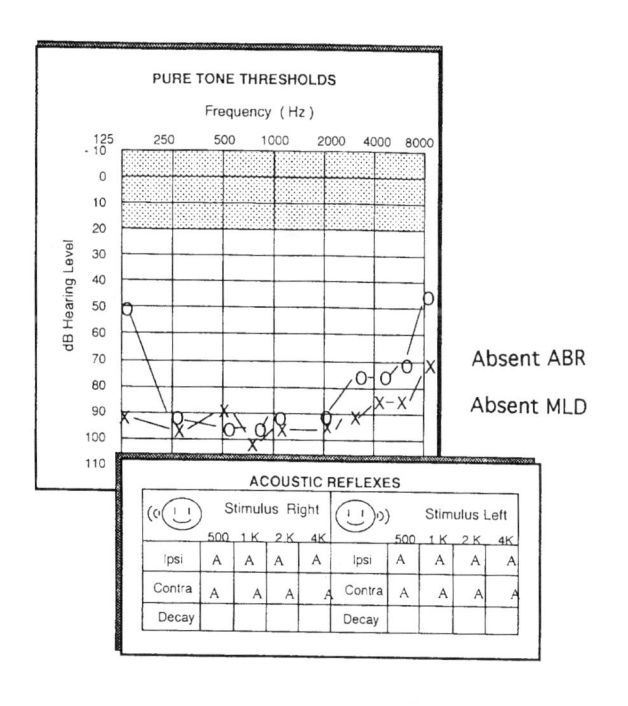

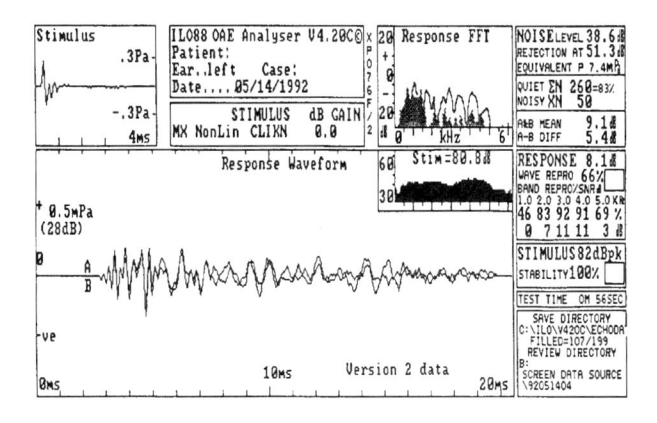

Figure 6–3. See Figure 6–2.

103

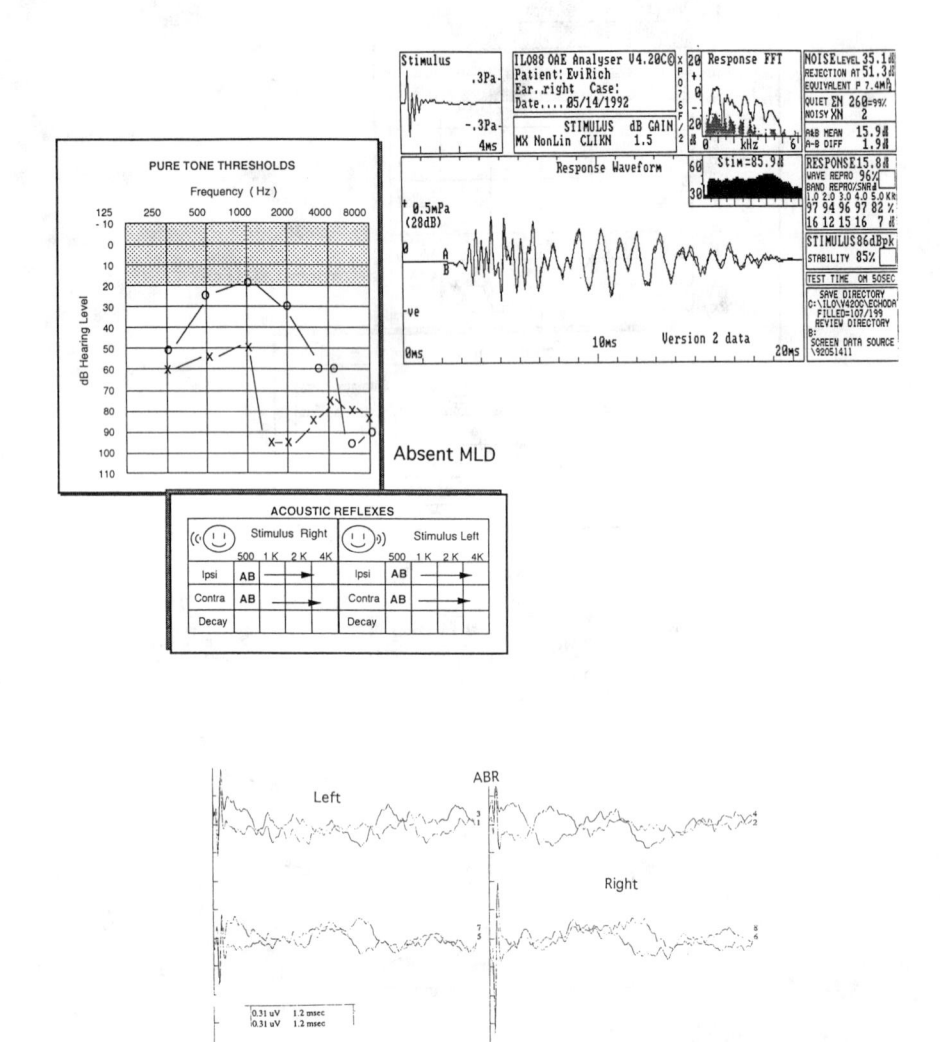

Figure 6–4. See Figure 6–2.

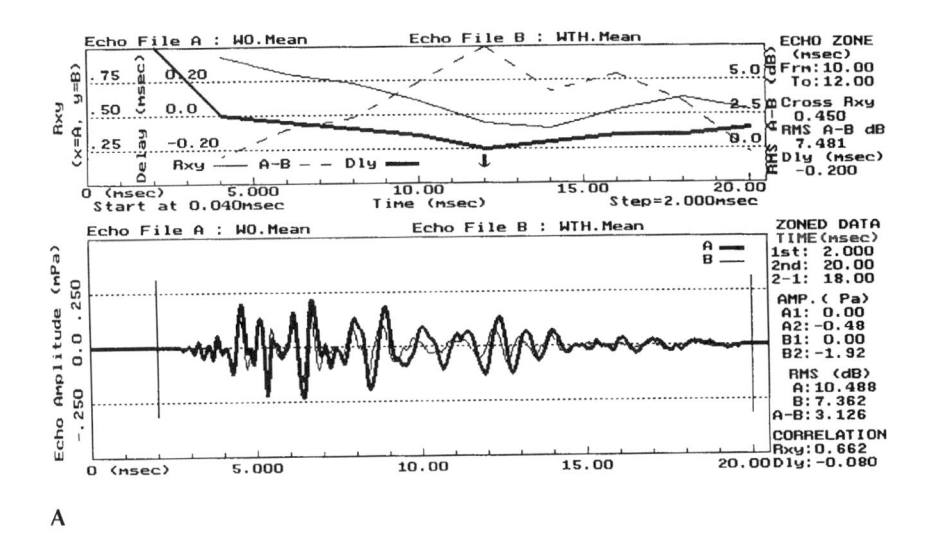

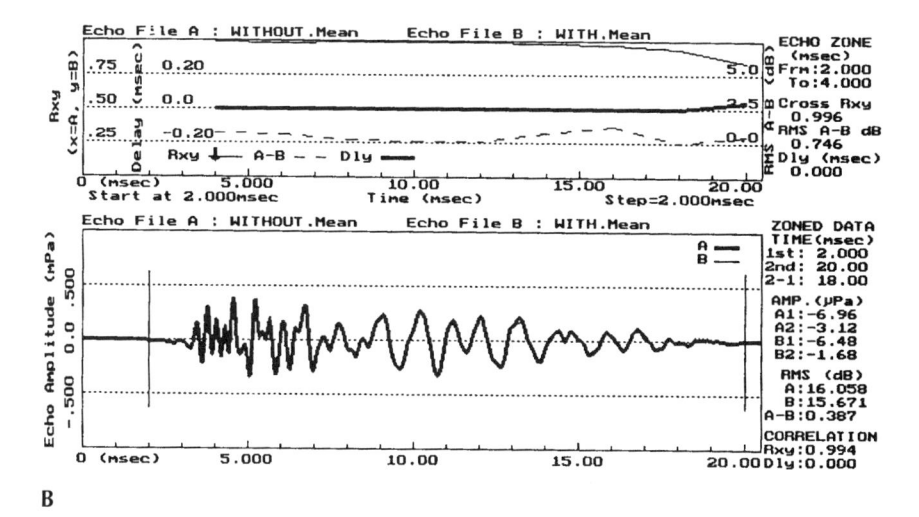

Figure 6–5. A: A typical click-evoked emission obtained from subjects with normal hearing. **B:** Three virtually parallel lines depicting the absence of suppression in all of the patients with auditory neuropathy.

for the measurements completed with Han Wen's Kresge Echomaster System (1993; Figure 6–5a). Figure 6–5b comes from a patient with auditory neuropathy and shows the pathologic three parallel lines common to all of these patients when studied by efferent suppression techniques. Clearly the nature of their pure tone audiograms is misleading with respect to hearing aid need or success.

Patient 1

This patient was sent to us as part of our search for Ultra-audiometric subjects (Berlin et al., 1978). Her rising audiogram (Figure 6–6) suggested

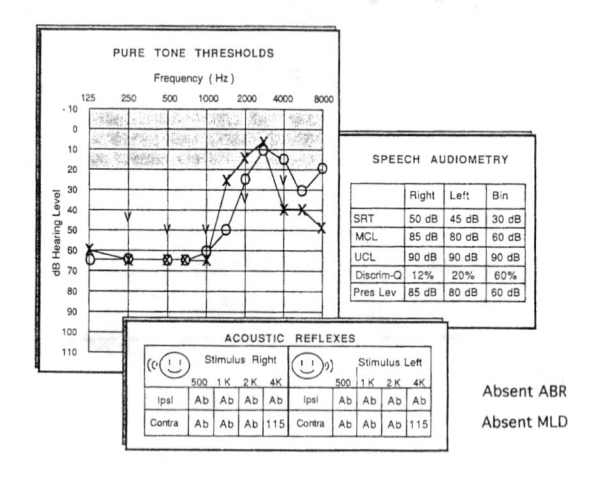

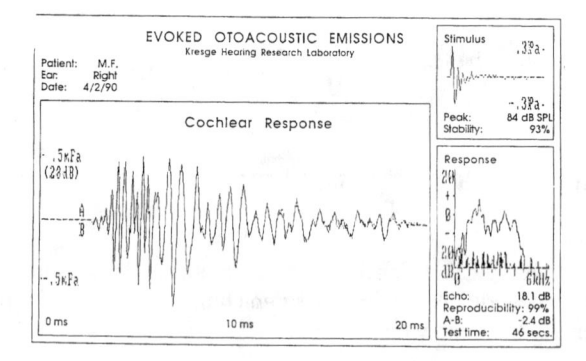

Figure 6–6. Patient with auditory neuropathy and low frequency loss who also has no ABR, no MLD, but normal otoacoustic emissions.

she would be an excellent candidate for hearing aids of one of two types—either a low-frequency emphasis aid with no insertion loss (Killion, Berlin, & Hood, 1984) or one of our body borne translators (Berlin et al., 1978). Her clinical complaint was that she simply could not understand speech in quiet or in noise, and also suffered from mild unsteadiness and poor coordination. She manages quite well in everyday life with the help of her husband, and runs a successful service business. We were not sophisticated enough at the time to recognize the signs that she was not a candidate for ordinary amplification. She tried the K-Bass (Killion et al., 1984) aid with the report that it helped heighten her awareness that someone was talking to her but it did not help her understand speech. We were puzzled at the time over the **absence** of an ABR to clicks or tone bursts around 2 kHz and sent her for a neurological workup. She was diagnosed as having an unspecified leukodystrophy, not MS, and has had no further clarification of her status since then, other than her disease resembles Charcot-Marie-Tooth syndrome but is slightly different (Starr & Picton, personal communication).

Audiological Findings

Her middle ear muscle reflexes were absent despite normal tympanometry. Also absent were any release from masking during MLD testing (Hirsh, 1948) and any synchronous ABR discharge, either to clicks or tone bursts around the zone of her normal hearing. Most surprising, however, were her unusually large and spectrally complex otoacoustic emissions which conventional wisdom predicted would be absent except in a narrow zone between 2 and 3 kHz. (Figure 6–6).

She showed complete absence of contralateral suppression of her otoacoustic emissions at any combination of click intensities and noise levels we used (ranging from 60 to 80 dB peak SP). Because of the absence of both the first wave of the ABR and the total absence of efferent suppression, we conclude that the primary neurons are not synchronous enough to activate an efferent outflow from the brainstem (Berlin et al., 1994).

Patient 2

This 40-year-old woman came to us originally carrying a diagnosis of Charcot-Marie-Tooth syndrome passed down from her father. Her sister is similarly afflicted and, as a matter of fact, is the next patient in this chapter. Figure 6–3 shows her audiogram, and Figure 6–4 shows the somewhat less severe appearing pure tone loss of her sister. It is reasonable to anticipate that Patient 2 would not have much of an ABR, MLD, or middle ear muscle reflex. But what is surprising is that she has normal and robust otoacoustic emissions and absolutely no contralateral suppression. The evidence for her systemic neuropathy comes from the absence of sensory nerve response in her right arm, and slowed transmission time and reduced motor response of the right median nerve, with normal response of the ulnar nerve. She had no success with the hearing aids we had prescribed (before we observed her normal otoacoustic emissions data).

Patient 3

This 36-year-old woman, who is the sister of the previous patient, also shows no middle ear muscle reflexes, no ABR, no MLD, and large and robust otoacoustic emissions, a paradoxical finding again in view of her pure tone hearing loss (Figure 6–4). She too showed no contralateral suppression and had no success with any hearing aids we tried.

Patient 4

The first three patients all had abnormal audiograms for which one might prescribe hearing aids if one had no information about otoacoustic emissions. In stark contrast, Patient 4 has a nearly normal audiogram but no ABR, no middle ear muscle reflex response, and would have appeared to be deaf, if we had tested him only with ABRs (Figure 6–2). Since he was brought to us at age 12 with a complaint that he simply couldn't understand other people's speech, he was easy to test behaviorally. That's how we found that, despite his absent ABR, he had normal otoacoustic emissions, no efferent suppression, and no MLDs.

What Do the Outer Hair Cells Do?

Outer hair cells probably contribute to some form of mechanical or electrical amplification of low amplitude acoustic inputs or compression of high amplitude inputs. Among the most illuminating observations in this area are the Mossbauer studies (Ruggero, 1992) summarized in Figure 6–7. Here we see that for a 3 dB input signal at 9 kHz the hair cells reflect a 10,000× amplification. In contrast, when the input signal reaches 80 dB, the hair cells impart a little more than 10× amplification. It is clear that outer hair cells play an important part in whatever compression mechanisms operate in the normal ear. The gain functions of the K-Amp and ReSound hearing aids (Figure 6–8) are qualitatively similar to the gain functions Ruggero observed.

The key issue here is that linear amplification doesn't work very well with ordinary outer hair cell hearing losses. They require a nondistorting

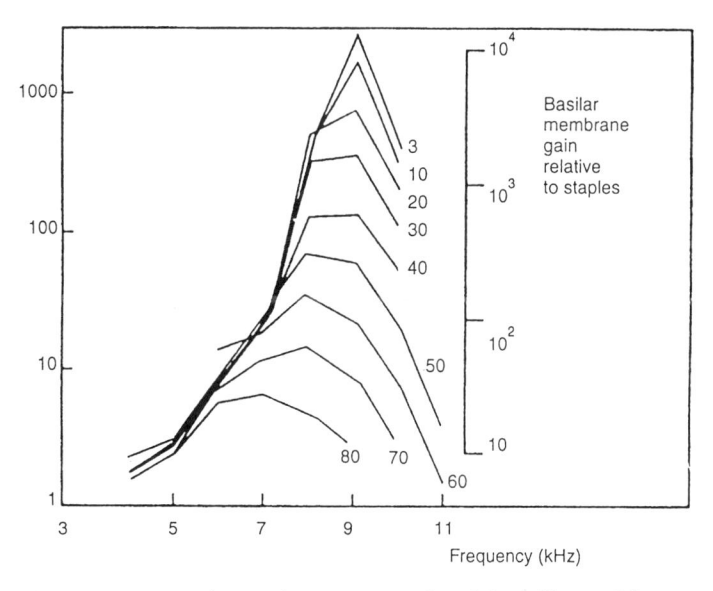

HEARING AIDS: ONLY FOR HEARING-IMPAIRED PATIENTS   **109**

Figure 6-7. Mechanical responses of a chinchilla cochlea to tones. Note that at peak, this gain is more than 10,000 for the lowest stimulus level (3 dB SPL) but drops to values between 10 and 100 for sound levels typical of speech (60 dB SPL to 80 dB SPL). Taken with permission from Ruggero (1992).

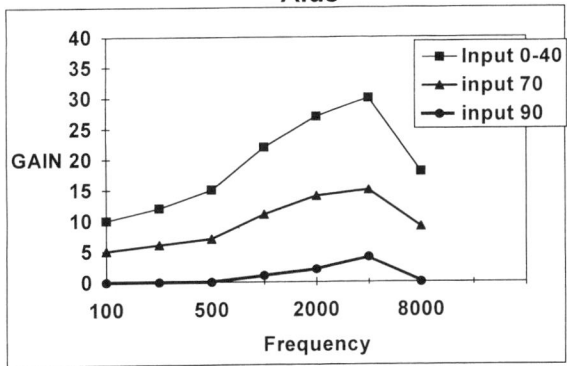

Figure 6-8. An idealized gain curve for K-Amp or dynamic compression programmable aids. Notice how these curves mimic the hair cell reducing gain functions shown in Figure 6-6.

decreasing gain system with increasing input which compensates for the disruptive effects of recruitment on the complex speech signal. It is this expansion of the loudness of vowel peaks and loss of perceived consonant-vowel relationships in speech that will be the topic of the next presentation (Villchur, 1973, 1974).

SUMMARY AND CONCLUSIONS

Otoacoustic emissions and ABR, when used together, form a powerful combination, offering insight into preneural as well as neural function in the cochlea. If emissions are present, patients are *not* hearing aid candidates. Conversely, it is the *absence* of outer hair cell echoes, in the presence of robust and synchronous ABRs at high intensities, that suggests that patients with hearing losses from 20 to 70 dB HL are *good* candidates for dynamic compression aids. These aids compensate for the presumed loss of the low-level amplification ascribed to the outer hair cells, which bring faint sounds into smooth, broad-band, audibility.

Unfortunately, many people are living today with "yesterday's diagnosis": *You have "nerve deafness" and hearing aids will be of limited value.* The fact is that linear aids with restricted frequency responses and ordinary peak clipping simply drove many patients to take the aids off. The aids made vocalic segments of speech disproportionately loud and hence distorted to the listener who was hearing impaired. Because of their restricted frequency response, these aids also limited the quality and number of auditory cues patients could use to hear both in noise and in crowds the way people with normal hearing do.

The kernel message: it is no longer appropriate to fit a linear hearing aid to patients with hair-cell-based losses from 20 to 75dB HL. High fidelity dynamic compression aids that make low-level signals uniformly and smoothly audible are useful answers to the sharp and uneven loudness growth of segments of the speech code for people with recruitment.

Acknowledgments: NIDCD Center Grant P0 1 DC-000379, Training Grants T32-DC-00007, Department of Defense Neuroscience Center Grant via N. Bazan, Kam's Fund for Hearing Research, The Kleberg Foundation, Lions' Eye Foundation and District 8-S Charities. Special support for the entire document and this chapter as well came from Dr. S. Singh, General Hearing Instruments, Etymotic Research, Dr. A. Lippa and Hearing Innovations, and NDIB-BMDR 1549.

REFERENCES

Berlin, C. I., Hood, L. J., Cecola, R. P., Jackson, D. F., & Szabo, P. (1993). Does Type I afferent neuron dysfunction reveal itself through lack of efferent suppression? *Hearing Research, 65*, 40–50.

Berlin, C. I., Hood, L. J., Hurley, A., & Wen, H. (1994). Contralateral suppression of otoacoustic emissions: An index of the function of the medial olivocochlear system. *Otolaryngology Head and Neck Surgery, 110*, 3–21.

Berlin, C. I., Hood, L. J., Wen, H., Szabo, P., Cecola, R. P., Rigby, P., & Jackson, D. F., (1993). Contralateral suppression of non-linear click evoked otoacoustic emissions. *Hearing Research, 71*, 1–11.

Berlin, C. I., Wexler, K. F., Jerger, J. F., Halperin, H. R., & Smith, S. (1978). Superior ultra-audiometric hearing: A new type of hearing loss which correlates highly with unusually good speech in the "profoundly deaf." *Otolaryngology, 86*, 111–116.

Hirsh, I. (1948). The influence of interaural phase on interaural summation and inhibition. *Journal of the Acoustical Society of America, 20*, 536–544.

Killion, M. C., Berlin, C. I., & Hood, L. J. (1984). A low frequency emphasis open-canal hearing aid. *Hearing Instruments, 35*, 30–34, 66.

Kujawa, S., Glattke, T. J., Fallon, M., & Bobbin, R. P. (1991). A nicotinic receptor mediates suppression of the distortion product otoacoustic emission by contralateral sound. *Hearing Research, 74*, 122–134.

Liberman, M. C. (1989). Response properties of cochlear efferent neurons; monaural vs. binaural stimulation and the effects of noise. *Journal of Neurophysiology, 60*, 1779–1798.

Puel, J-L., & Rebillard, G. (1990). Effect of contralateral sound stimulation on the distortion product 2 f1–f2: Evidence that the medial efferent system is involved. *Journal of the Acoustical Society of America, 87*, 1630–1635.

Ruggero, M. A. (1992). Responses to sound of the basilar membrane of mammalian cochlea. *Current Opinion Neurobiology, 2*, 449–456.

Sininger, Y., Hood, L. J., Starr, A., Berlin, C. I., & Picton, T. (1995). Hearing loss due to auditory neuropathy. *Audiology Today, 7*, 10–13.

Starr, A., McPherson, D., Patterson, J., Don, M., Luxford, W., Shannon, R., Sininger, Y., Tonokawa, L., & Waring, M. (1991). Absence of both auditory evoked potentials and auditory percepts dependent on time cues. *Brain, 114*, 1157–1180.

Villchur, E. (1973). Signal processing to improve speech intelligibility in perceptive deafness. *Journal of the Acoustical Society of America, 53*, 1646.

Villchur, E. (1974). Simulation of the effect of recruitment on loudness relationships in speech. *Journal of the Acoustical Society of America, 56*, 1601–1611.

Warr, W. B., Guinan, J. J., & White, J. S. (1986). Organization of the efferent fibers: The lateral and medial olivocochlear systems. In R. A. Altschuler, R. P. Bobbin, & D. W. Hoffman (Eds.), *Neurobiology of hearing: The cochlea* (pp. 333–348). New York: Raven Press.

Warr, W. B., & Guinan, J. J. (1978). Efferent innervation of the organ of Corti: Two different systems. *Brain Research, 173*, 152–155.

7

Multichannel Compression in Hearing Aids

Edgar Villchur
Foundation for Hearing Aid Research,
Woodstock, New York

INTRODUCTION

It is a special source of satisfaction in science when the results of research in one discipline coincide with the results of research in another discipline. That is what has happened here: The analyses and studies we have been listening to on the physiology of the inner ear, and of the functions of the hair cells, lead to the same conclusions that were reached by researchers in audiology working with data from subject responses.

RECRUITMENT

In the 1930s audiological researchers discovered a phenomenon they called *recruitment*, the progressive alleviation of hearing impairment as the input level of sound increases. A person with recruitment may be very deaf to weak sounds and progressively less deaf to more intense sounds, until, in cases of "complete" recruitment, at some high level the listener with impaired hearing has the same loudness response as that of a listener with normal hearing.

Recruitment was first referred to by E. P. Fowler in the *Archives of Otolaryngology* (1936), and a few months later Steinberg and Gardner published a paper on recruitment in the *Journal of the Acoustical Society of America* (1937). But it was Steinberg and Gardner who understood the implications of recruitment for amplification for hearing-impaired persons. If you provide enough amplification for a person with recruitment to make the weak sounds of speech audible, the same amount of amplification applied to intense sounds is likely to drive the listener out of his or her skull. It may be for that reason that recruitment is often referred to—inaccurately—as an abnormal intolerance for intense sound. That description only applies when you overamplify; recruitment actually has its greatest effect on the weakest sounds.

The discovery of recruitment had an obvious implication for hearing aids, one that Steinberg and Gardner described in their prophetic 1937 paper: "Owing to the expanding action of this type of loss, it would be necessary to introduce a corresponding compression in the amplifier" (p. 20). Fowler (1942), on the other hand, thought of recruitment as an ameliorating factor in hearing impairment. In an article on the calculation of the "percent" of hearing loss for compensation cases, he suggested that for up to 40 dB of loss, the recruitment factor ought to reduce the calculated percent of loss.

AMPLITUDE COMPRESSION TO COMPENSATE FOR RECRUITMENT

Caraway and Carhart (1967) subjected speech to amplitude compression in an attempt to improve speech understanding for hearing-impaired subjects by compensating for their recruitment. They used a three-channel compressor but offered no rationale for the use of more than one channel (Caraway told me they had ordered a compressor and it had come with three channels, each channel with identical processing characteristics.) They did not use frequency-response shaping in combination with the compression, which we will see is as important as the compression; and they made no processing adjustments between one subject and the next. The results were negative. What Caraway and Carhart succeeded in demonstrating, I think, was that a compressor used as a black box between the signal and the subject, rather than as part of a flexible signal-processing system designed to match and compensate for the individual hearing aberrations of the subject, is not likely to improve speech understanding.

In 1973 I reported a study in the *Journal of the Acoustical Society of America* in which a two-channel compressor was included in a speech-processing system for hearing-impaired subjects. The first step in the experiment was to map out the residual frequency and dynamic range of hearing of each subject. Figure 7–1 is a diagram of the average residual dynamic range of hearing for speech, over most of the frequency spectrum, of the six subjects of that study. I define this residual dynamic range of hearing as the area bracketed by (1) the impaired threshold and

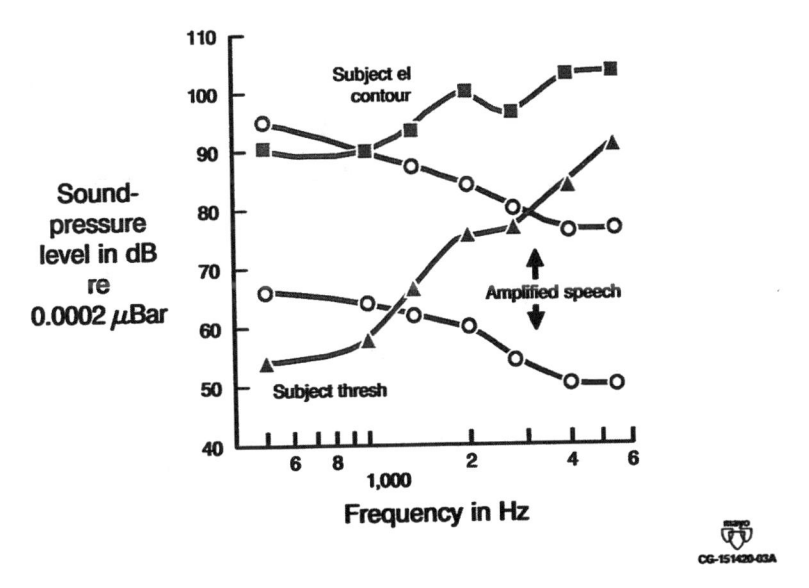

Figure 7–1. Average residual dynamic range of hearing of the six subjects of the Villchur study of 1973 and the proportionate positions of amplified speech levels relative to that dynamic range. The dynamic range of hearing for speech is defined as the area between hearing threshold and an equal-loudness contour anchored at 1 kHz to the preferred level for listening to speech (from Villchur, 1974).

(2) a measured equal-loudness contour anchored at 1 kHz to the preferred level for listening to amplified speech. (The curves in Figure 7–1 are averages, but the processing for each subject was based on individual measurements.) Plotted against this residual dynamic range of hearing is the frequency/amplitude band of conversational speech as measured by Dunn and White (1940) in half-octave bands. The speech band is shown amplified to the average preferred level of the six subjects when listening to speech.

Although the speech has been amplified without distortion to the preferred level of the subject, a large portion of it lies below the threshold of hearing, which is to say it is inaudible. This inaudible portion of the speech is where the high-frequency consonants, which are extremely important as intelligence-bearing elements, occur.

To put the diagram of Figure 7–1 into perspective, Figure 7–2 shows the normal dynamic range of hearing for speech, between normal threshold and the 74-phon equal-loudness contour. Plotted against this normal dynamic range is the unamplified frequency/amplitude range of conver-

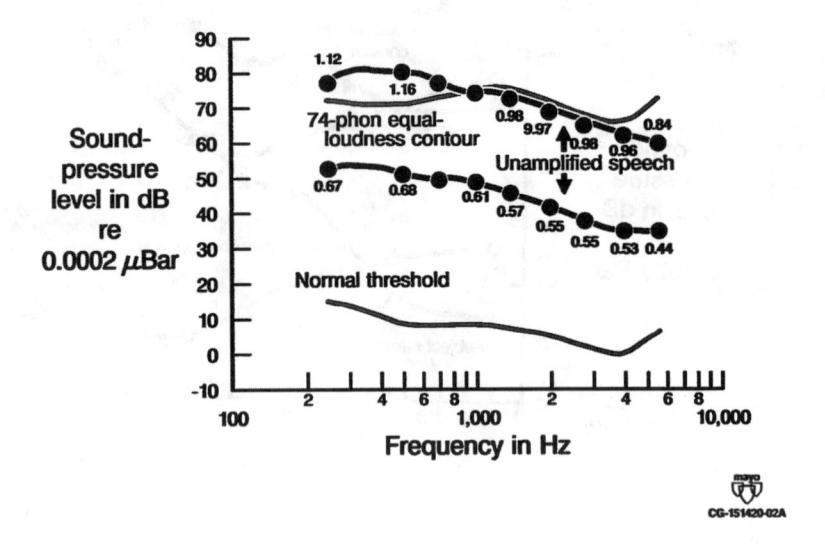

Figure 7–2. Proportionate positions of unamplified conversational speech levels relative to the dynamic range between the normal threshold of hearing and the ISO 74-phon equal-loudness contour (from Villchur, 1973).

sational speech measured by Dunn and White; the 74-phon contour was chosen for Figure 7–2 because it intersects the high-amplitude contour of the Dunn-White speech band at 1 kHz. Dunn and White reported that the limitations of their 1940 equipment prevented them from measuring the lowest 20% or so of speech levels, but even if we lower the bottom line of speech levels another 20%, it is evident that the weakest elements of speech lie well above normal threshold.

It does not take a rocket scientist to determine what needs to be done to the speech in Figure 7–1 to make it fit into the residual dynamic range of hearing in such a way that all elements will be audible. We need to squeeze the speech band vertically, which is to say subject it to amplitude compression, more at high frequencies than at low frequencies because it has to fit into a narrower channel (this is one reason a separate compressor is used for the high-frequency region). Then we need to bend the speech band upward, which is to say give it high-frequency emphasis, so that the compressed speech takes its proper position in the high-frequency region of the residual dynamic range of hearing of the subject.

Figure 7–3 shows that being done: The processed speech now fits fairly well. The elements of speech that were inaudible are now audible.

MULTICHANNEL COMPRESSION IN HEARING AIDS 117

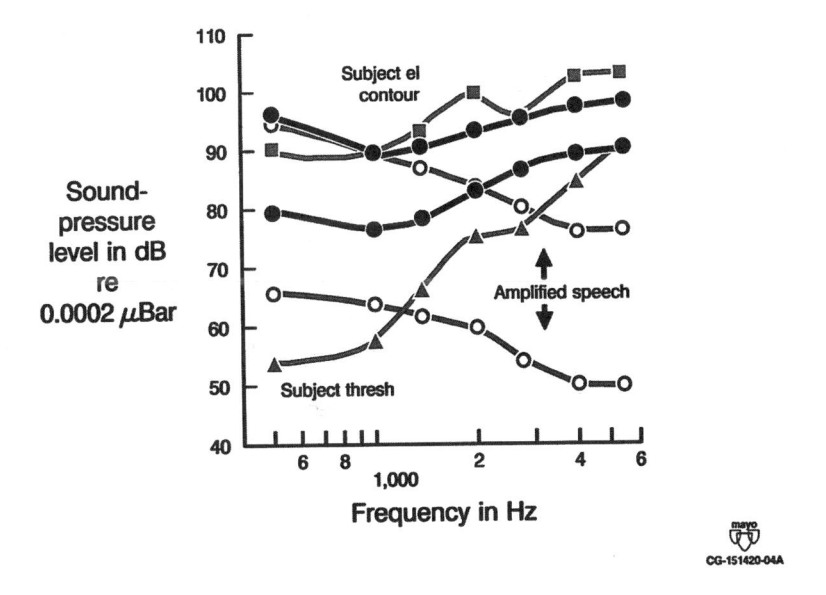

Figure 7–3. Effect of subjecting speech to compression and frequency-response shaping. The processed speech has approximately the same position relative to the residual dynamic range of hearing as the unamplified speech of Figure 7–2 relative to the normal dynamic range.

Vincent Pluvinage, who was a member of the Bell Laboratories team (led by the late Fred Waldhauer) that converted the rack-mounted equipment of my 1973 experiment to a 1.4 volt chip suitable for a wearable hearing aid, has described this processing in audiological terms rather than the acoustical terms I have used here. The gain for a linear hearing aid is often calculated in terms of a "gain rule," which is the gain at a particular frequency expressed as a percentage of the threshold hearing loss at that frequency. Pluvinage points out that with linear amplification it is necessary to choose a compromise gain rule, one that provides too much gain for the high-amplitude elements of speech and not enough gain for the low-amplitude elements of speech. A compressor system, on the other hand, provides an adaptive gain rule that increases for the lower speech levels.

Using Pluvinage's approach, I calculated the gain rules used in Figure 7–3 at 3 kHz. The gain rule required to lift the highest-amplitude elements of speech at this frequency to their proper levels in the processed speech is 37%. The gain rule required to lift the lowest-amplitude elements of speech to their proper levels in the processed speech is 67%.

THE PHYSIOLOGICAL BASIS OF RECRUITMENT

We can talk about compression processing from a third point of view, that of physiology. The extra gain provided by compression for the weaker sounds is an electronic substitute for the lost function of the outer hair cells. In Chapter 1, William Brownell described the action of the outer hair cells as amplifiers for the inner hair cells. The outer hair cells do not merely respond passively to sound stimuli, they amplify it, which is to say they inject additional energy into the system. Charles Berlin pointed out that the outer hair cells provide a large amount of amplification for weak signals and only a small amount of amplification for intense signals. They are level-dependent amplifiers. It is the outer hair cells that are lost first in hearing impairment, causing recruitment; electronic compression in the hearing aid (level-dependent amplification) replaces the physiological compression that has been lost. The apparent "expanding action" of recruitment referred to by Steinberg and Gardner is actually a loss of the normal compressor action of the outer hair cells.

RESEARCH ON NOISE SUPPRESSION

Research in signal processing for hearing aids after 1973 was mainly of two types: research on compression and research on noise suppression. It was known that hearing-impaired persons find it especially difficult to understand speech in noise, and it was also known that hearing aids didn't seem to help. Tillman, Carhart, and Olsen (1970) showed that hearing aids of their day actually made things worse, in the sense that the wearer needed a better signal-to-noise ratio to understand speech with the hearing aid than without it. These hearing aids not only failed to restore speech cues the subject could no longer hear, but the poor quality of their amplification reduced the number of cues the subject could hear. And so it seemed logical to try to design an electronic circuit that would suppress the noise relative to the speech. Closer examination shows this approach is not as logical as it seems.

Consider a computer-controlled electronic circuit that can separate the voices of several people talking at the same time, or at least favor one over the others. Such a circuit would have to respond to identifying cues such as voice quality, speech mannerisms, and the meaningful sequences of syllables and words; it would have to know not to combine syllables and words of one talker with the syllables and words of another. A very powerful computer and complex program is called for, one that is clearly impractical for a hearing aid. Yet the most common "noise" with which hearing-impaired persons must contend is just such competing speech.

But we don't have to give up hope. Such a computer and program do exist; the computer is portable, and we all own one. It is the computer in the human brain. Broadbent (1958) described the ability of humans to listen selectively; we can pay attention to a particular message among simultaneous competing messages. We can do what a hearing aid computer cannot, because we have the necessary information in our memory banks—including a knowledge of the language—and a powerful computing capacity. Mead Killion (1993) has pointed out that the most powerful computer in the world can recognize a human face in half an hour, but a baby can do it in half a second.

The attention mechanism is central rather than sensory, and therefore requires that the target message be recognizable; we listen selectively by picking out recognizable patterns, or Gestalts, from the total sound. How, then, do we overcome the masking effect of competing signals on the target speech? We do it by taking advantage of the redundancy of speech cues. Coker (1974) called speech an error-resistant code because the code contains many redundant cues to its meaning. For example, speech that is cut off sharply above 2 kHz is readily understandable, but so is speech that is cut off *below* 2 kHz. The redundant cues of speech provide a reserve against the loss of cues to masking, and make it possible for listeners with normal hearing to understand speech in a high-noise environment. But listeners who are hearing impaired do not hear many of the speech cues, even after undistorted amplification. The part of the speech they do hear may be enough for understanding speech in quiet, but when the impoverished set of cues available to them suffers a further loss from masking, there are insufficient redundant cues left for them to fall back on.

All of this brings us back to the subject discussed earlier, signal processing to restore elements of speech that, even after linear amplification, remain inaudible to the impaired listener because of recruitment and high-frequency loss. The importance of restoring acoustical speech cues to the residual hearing of subjects is increased when they are listening in noise. Circuits designed to suppress noise typically go the other way: They sacrifice rather than restore speech cues.

A few years ago I looked up my 1973 paper in the *Journal of the Acoustical Society of America* relative to this noise problem, and I found something I hadn't noticed earlier. Table 7–1 shows average intelligibility scores from that study. The upper table represents the average scores of all six subjects under three conditions: linear amplification with voice interference, linear amplification with the interference removed, and compression/equalization amplification with the interference put back in. The lower table lists the average scores of the three subjects who were most severely impaired. The scores are rearranged from the way they

TABLE 7-I. *Upper Table:* average speech-recognition scores (percent phonemes correct in CVC nonsense syllables) of six hearing-impaired subjects under three conditions (from Villchur, 1973). *Lower Table:* average scores of the three most severely impaired subjects. Leaving out the interference in Column 2 is the equivalent of adding an ideal noise suppressor to the linear amplification of speech-plus-interference represented in Column 1.

	Linear		Compressed/equalized
	Voice interference at -10 dB	Interference removed	Voice interference at -10 dB
Initial consonant	48.2%	60.0	63.2
Vowel	70.7	77.0	83.3
Terminal consonant	34.0	40.3	49.0
Initial consonant	32.7%	52.7	57.6
Vowel	59.0	72.0	79.3
Terminal consonant	25.7	31.3	43.6

% phonemes correct

were presented in 1973: The original reference was the column of scores for linear amplification in quiet.

It should come as no surprise that the recognition scores in the second column, for linear amplification in quiet, are higher than the scores in the first column, for linear amplification in noise. But it may come as something of a surprise that the scores in the third column, representing processed amplification in noise, are actually higher than the scores for linear amplification in quiet. When listening in noise, these subjects benefitted more from compression/equalization processing than they did from the equivalent of a perfect and unachievable noise suppressor, one that eliminates the noise and leaves the speech unaffected. (All of the speech-in-noise scores were improved by the processing, but only four of the six were higher than the scores in quiet.)

To illustrate that speech understanding in noise can be increased even though the relative noise is greater, simulations of the two most common hearing pathologies, recruitment and accentuated high-frequency loss, are included on the CD that accompanies this book. Electronic simulations have a special function: They make it possible to isolate particular pathologies in the simulation, and to judge whether that pathology has a significant effect on speech understanding. Remember that Fowler thought recruitment was an advantage at some levels.

The simulation was made with a bank of electronic expanders to simulate the recruitment, and a low-pass filter to simulate the high-frequency loss. These were not used blindly, but were adjusted to represent a particular subject's hearing characteristics. In 1974 I published an article on such a simulation, with a plastic record bound in, that included a report on an experiment to validate the simulation[1]. Later I used simulation equipment with a larger number of channels; the tape we will hear today was made with a 12-channel simulator, built by my good friend and colleague Mead Killion of Etymotic Research.

The first band is of speech with voice interference, simulating the loudness relationships heard by a subject with severe recruitment and high-frequency loss, listening through a linear hearing aid (Track 0001).

The next band is of the same speech and interference affected by the same hearing pathologies, but here the simulation is of the loudness relationships the subject would hear through a properly adjusted compression/equalization hearing aid (Track 0002). The compensation processing I used in 1974 had to be done with laboratory equipment; there were no hearing aids then that could do that job. The present simulation was done with the electronics of a Resound hearing aid. I chose a Resound because its basic design is very close to that of my original rack-mounted laboratory compression/equalization equipment.

The relative level of the interference in this last band was increased by the compression, but many listeners do not notice it because they are distracted by the increased clarity of the target speech.

It is possible to provide effective improvement in the signal-to-noise ratio by acoustical rather than electronic means. Directional microphones, or microphones placed at the talker rather than the listener position (an effective but inconvenient procedure), can reduce the relative level of interference without compromising the speech signal.

---

[1]Although we cannot know exactly what such a subject hears, we can feel reasonably confident of the accuracy of simulation of at least one element, the loudness relationships among speech elements. This type of expansion/equalization simulation was validated (Villchur, 1974) by having subjects with only one impaired ear compare the simulation in the good ear with the real thing, amplified to the same loudness, in the impaired ear.

COMPRESSION RESEARCH OF THE 1970s AND 1980s

At least half the compression research after 1973 came to the conclusion that compression was not the way to go. One of the reasons for some of these negative results, I believe, had to do with the test material used in the studies. It had been standard procedure to use speech tests that were recorded by a talker facing a VU meter, reading single-syllable words, and carefully keeping all words at the same level. Many investigators used the same kind of speech tests in their compression experiments, so that in effect the linear reference for their speech tests was precompressed by a human compressor. For example, O'Loughlin (1980) published a study using such single-syllable speech material, and in order to increase the dynamic range of his material he presented the tests at three levels separated by 10 dB each. The levels were not varied, however, until *after* the compression, so that the compressor was never given the opportunity to operate on the change of levels.

Plomp (1988) published a paper in which he stated that theoretical considerations predict that the kind of compression I have been describing reduces speech understanding for both listeners with normal hearing and listeners with impaired hearing. He said that compression reduces intensity contrasts, or fluctuations of the wave envelope, and since this distorts the speech it necessarily reduces intelligibility. It is entirely true that compression reduces intensity contrasts in speech—just as the action of the outer hair cells reduces the intensity contrasts in the signals stimulating the inner hair cells—but if the compression and equalization are properly adjusted to compensate for the impairment of the subject, the processing restores the *loudness* relationships in speech to normal. If the wave envelope of the compressed speech were plotted in units of loudness rather than intensity, the compressed envelope would not appear distorted but rather normal or close to normal. Plomp fell back to the position that recruitment failed to reduce the just noticeable difference (jnd) for intensity, although we would expect it to, and this implies that compression would increase the jnd for intensity. While this is true, I do not know of any evidence that the size of the jnd is significant to speech understanding. My response to Plomp's theoretical objections appeared in the same journal in 1989.

Today there is still a rear-guard action being fought against compression. Many hearing aid manufacturers use compression in at least some of their models, but the old idea of compression as a way of limiting high-level sound, with linear amplification employed up to some high level, seems to have a lingering influence. As far as I know only a few current hearing aids are properly classified as full-dynamic-range compression hearing aids, whose thresholds of compression are set at the levels of the weakest elements of speech. The thresholds of compression of the other compression aids are placed either at the middle of the dynamic range of speech or at the upper end.

CONCLUSION

I believe the key to successful compression/equalization processing is the accuracy with which the electronic compensation matches the characteristics of the hearing impairment. This processing has three necessary elements: more than one full-dynamic-range compression channel, to compensate for the varying degree of recruitment in different frequency regions (the K-AMP design achieves similar results in a different way), and to allow simultaneous independent compression in different channels; post-compression equalization, or frequency-response shaping; and the capability to adjust the processing characteristics to match the hearing impairment of each subject.

The discoveries discussed in this book provide a physiological basis for the audiological phenomenon of recruitment. Compensation for recruitment by compression turns out to be an electronic substitute for the physiological compression of the outer hair cells.

REFERENCES

Broadbent, D. E. (1958). *Perception and communication.* New York: Pergamon.

Caraway, B. J., & Carhart, R. (1967). Influence of compressor action on speech intelligibility, *Journal of the Acoustical Society of America, 41,* 1424–1433.

Coker, C. H. (1974). Speech as an error-resistant digital code, *Journal of the Acoustical Society of America, 55,* 476(A).

Dunn, H. K., & White, S. D. (1940). Statistical measurements on conversational speech, *Journal of the Acoustical Society of America, 11,* 277–288.

Fowler, E. P. (1936). A method for the early detection of otosclerosis, *Archives of Otolaryngology, 24,* 731–741.

Fowler, E. P. (1942). A simple method of measuring percentage of capacity for hearing speech, *Archives of Otolaryngology, 36,* 874–889.

Killion, M. C. (1993). The K-Amp hearing aid: An attempt to present high fidelity for persons with impaired hearing, *American Journal of Audiology, 2,* 52–74.

O'Loughlin, B. J. (1980). Evaluation of a three-channel compression amplification system on hearing-impaired children, *Australian Journal of Audiology, 2,* 1–9.

Plomp. R. (1988). The negative effect of amplitude compression in multichannel hearing aids in the light of the modulation transfer function, *Journal of the Acoustical Society of America, 83,* 2322–2327.

Steinberg, J. C., & Gardner, M. B. (1937). The dependence of hearing impairment on sound intensity, *Journal of the Acoustical Society of America, 9*, 11–23.

Tillman, T. W., Carhart, R., & Olsen, W. O. (1970). Hearing aid efficiency in a competing speech situation, *Journal of Speech and Hearing Research, 13*, 789-811.

Villchur, E. (1973). Signal processing to improve speech intelligibility in perceptive deafness, *Journal of the Acoustical Society of America, 53*, 1646–1657.

Villchur, E. (1974). Simulation of the effect of recruitment on loudness relationships in speech, *Journal of the Acoustical Society of America, 56*, 1601–1611. (Recording bound in with article.)

Villchur, E. (1989). Comments on "The negative effect of amplitude compression in multichannel hearing aids in the light of the modulation transfer function," *Journal of the Acoustical Society of America, 86*, 425–427 (L).

8

TALKING HAIR CELLS: WHAT THEY HAVE TO SAY ABOUT HEARING AIDS

Mead C. Killion, Ph.D.
President, Etymotic Research, 61 Martin Lane,
Elk Grove Village, IL 60007
Phone 708 228-0006 Fax 708 228-6836

When I submitted the title to this talk, I hoped that I would be able to play a demonstration of the ear talking. I didn't succeed in that, but I do have a demonstration of the ear playing music.

Thus I will begin by describing a method for "playing by ear"—using music by two famous composers to demonstrate this entertaining but meaningful use for otoacoustic emissions—and then discuss the changes in physiology and loudness growth accompanying three types of hearing loss. Different hearing losses require different hearing aid characteristics, which can now be chosen with increasingly solid theoretical justification. This leads to a discussion of loudness growth data and a brief discussion of individual differences in loudness growth and the repeatability of loudness measures.

TARTINI & BACH: PLAYING BY EAR
(THE HAIR CELLS PERFORM)

Figure 8–1 illustrates the generation of a Tartini tone. Tartini was a violinist back in the 1700s who is often credited with being the first to describe what violinists call the Tartini tones. If you simultaneously play the notes C and E on the A and E strings of a violin, for example, you will hear the

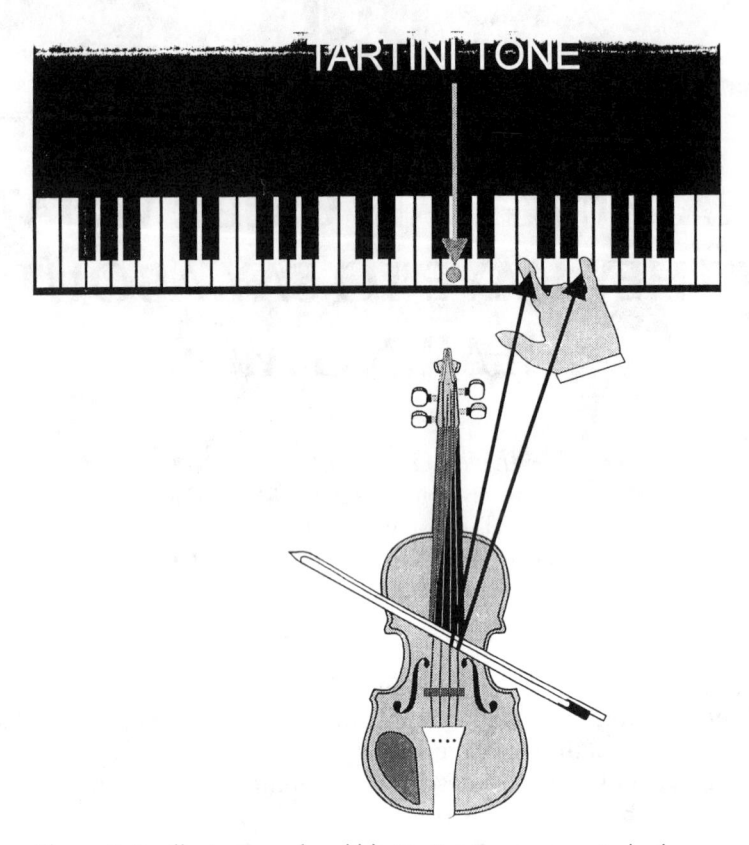

Figure 8–1. Illustration of audible Tartini Tone generated when a violin is played "double stop."

note G as illustrated in the figure.[1] The extra tone you hear—the same one violinists have been noticing for centuries—is the tone we are now measuring objectively in the earcanal. The difference is that now we call it the "cubic distortion product" tone at the frequency 2f1-f2 rather than the Tartini tone.

In the previous example, where f1 = 1047 Hz (C two octaves above middle C) and f2 = 1319 Hz (E), the cubic distortion tone is at the frequen-

---

[1]Checking this example out on a violin while this manuscript was being prepared, the author realized that the Tartini tone chosen for the sake of illustration was not the easiest one to hear. A better example might have been any of the pairs of notes he regularly plays on a piano to check out intermodulation distortion in hearing aids: The musical fourth C_5 and F_5 produces an audible note F_4 if the aid distorts badly. Similarly, B_4 and F_5 produce D_4; Bb_4 and F_5 produce Bb_3; A_4 and F_5 produce F3. (C_4 is middle C in this annotation.)

cy 2f1-f2 = 775 Hz (G). In point of fact, the frequency of 775 Hz is about 20 cents, or 1/5 of a semitone, below the musical note G. Many of the Tartini tones do not fall exactly on a note of the musical scale, which may have been what called them to Tartini's attention in the first place.

Just as Tartini tones are the products of intermodulation distortion in the ear, any nonlinear system exhibiting "cubic law" nonlinearity will generate Tartini tones. (Traditional starved-Class-A hearing aid amplifiers, for example, generate Tartini tones, although in hearing aids such tones are usually called intermodulation-distortion or cubic-distortion products.) In the past, it was difficult to provide a violinist with satisfactory hearing aids: the 105–115 dB SPL input on the violin side of the head created intermodulation distortion products much stronger than normal aural Tartini tones, making the violin nearly unplayable because the distortion from the hearing aid interfered with intonation.

In honor of Tartini, I should like to play a short recording from his Violin Sonata in G, the portion shown in Figure 8–2. The passage of music starting at circle C is the "Devil's Trill," a difficult section requiring two of the violinist's fingers to play the melody while the other two are engaged in a trill. According to Tartini, the Devil himself appeared at the foot of Tartini's bed in a dream one night in Assisi in 1713, playing the now-famous Devil's Trill on Tartini's own violin. (The section of music shown in Figure 8–2 was played for the attendees. It is Band 3 on the enclosed CD.)

Figure 8–3 shows the basic approach to "playing music by ear." One simply chooses successive pairs of frequencies that will generate each of the desired notes as Tartini tones. In the example shown, the desired note is an F, generated as the cubic distortion product of Bb and D. To make these recordings, we held Bb constant as f1 (using an oscillator, not a piano, of course), and then chose the value of f2 to produce the desired resultant tone. The data shown in Figures 8–3 to 8–5 were obtained with the aid of a low-noise ER-10C otoacoustic emissions probe sealed into the earcanal and the CUB^{e}DIS^{TM} analysis system (Allen, 1990). The CUB^{e}DIS system uses a synchronous averaging technique so that 4 seconds of averaging produces an equivalent 0.25 Hz bandwidth. The ER-10C uses a separate earphone driver for f1 and f2 to avoid the possibility of intermodulation distortion generated by the probe itself, and uses two microphones whose averaged output minimizes the noise level of the probe pickup.

As shown in Figure 8–4, as the frequency of f2 is increased, the frequency of the cubic distortion tone will decrease. The data shown in Figure 8–4 were obtained from the ear of Tim Monroe, a 27 year old male engineer with normal hearing and good aural emissions. Although there is a limit to the usable tones that can be produced with f1 = Bb, quite a few of the cubic distortion tones show a level of 5–10 dB SPL. These can

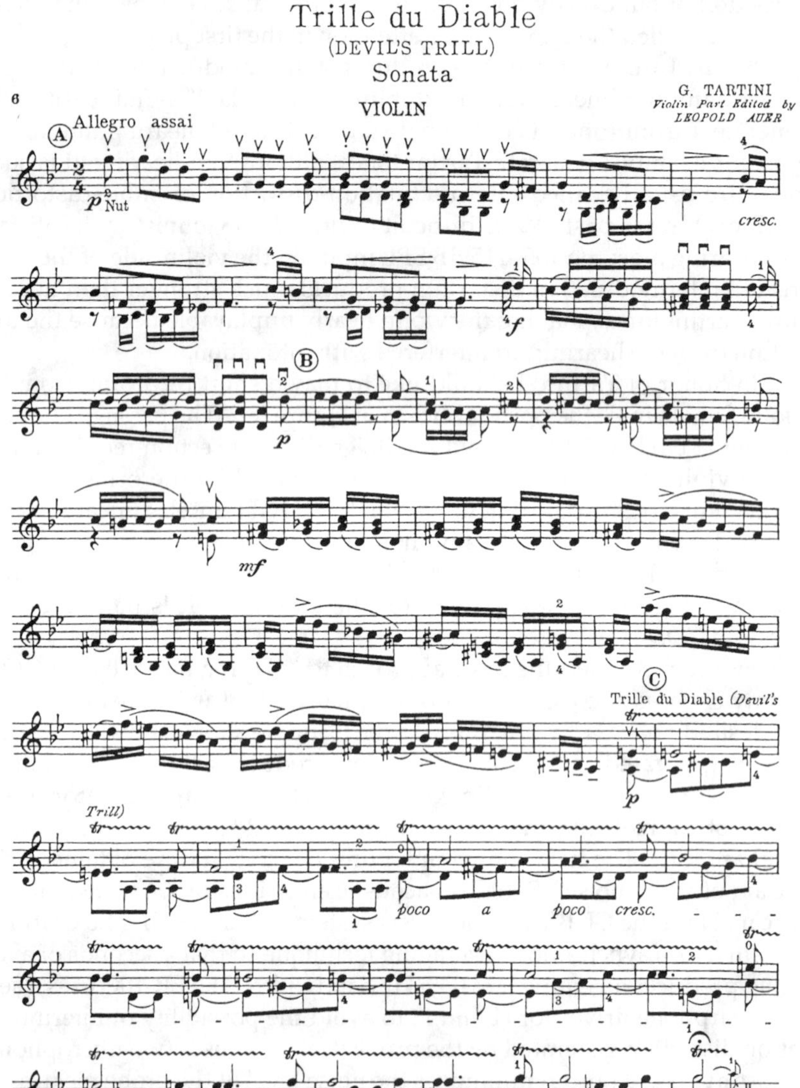

Figure 8–2. Portion of Tartini's Sonata in G.

GENERATION OF MUSIC NOTE F
AS CUBIC DISTORTION TONE FROM COMBINATION OF NOTES Bb AND D

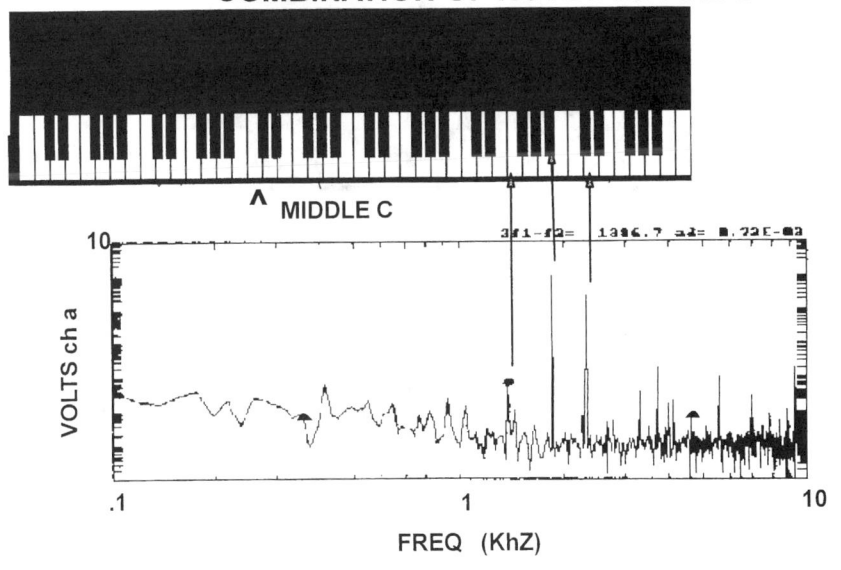

Figure 8–3. Generation of music note F played—literally—by ear. Note: In these figures, the piano keyboard has been scaled and positioned to line up with the frequency axis on the graph. The lowest octave on the piano—extending down to 27.5 Hz—has been omitted.

be heard without signal averaging, for the reasons discussed in the following paragraph.

The minimum pressure audible at the eardrum is about 12 dB SPL, so tones from the ear would be audible *directly* only if they exceeded 12 dB SPL.[2] By using a microphone quieter than the ear, however, tones below 12 dB can be detected and made audible by amplification. The internal noise of the ER-10C microphone, for example, has a spectrum level of about –20 dB SPL. The apparent bandwidth of the ear as a filter in this frequency region is roughly 100 Hz, based on the masking data of French & Steinberg (1947), who reported that a tone 18–22 dB above spectrum level is just audible to the average ear in the 1000–2500 Hz frequen-

---

[2] A good single-number approximation to the minimum audible pressure at the eardrum is 12 dB SPL; between 500 and 4000 Hz it lies within 3 dB of that value (Killion, 1978).

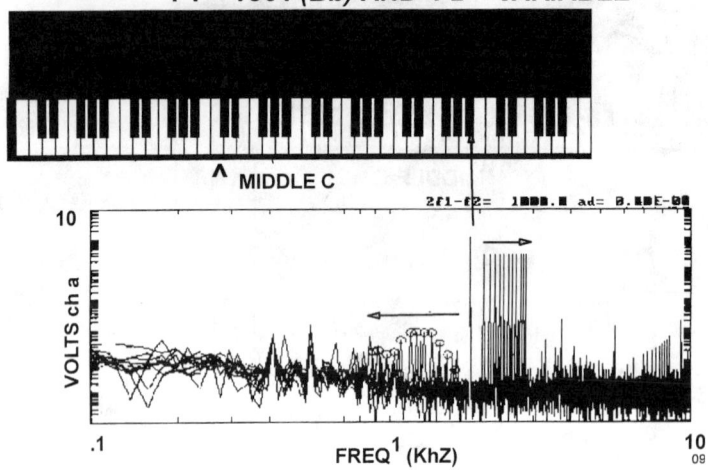

Figure 8–4. Generation of series of tones played by ear (Tim Monroe's).

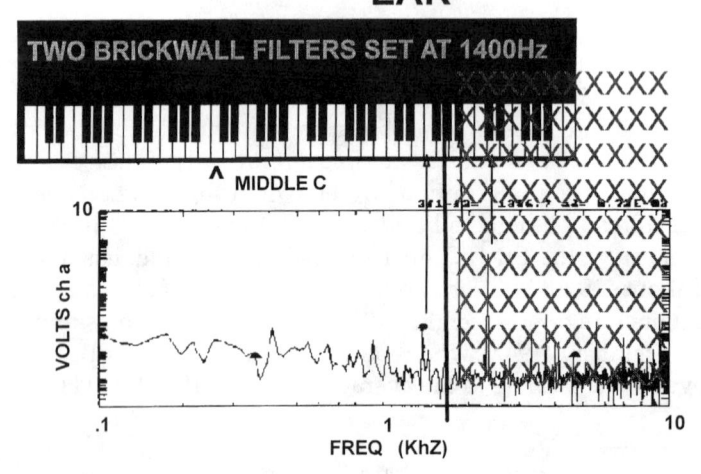

Figure 8–5. Use of two brick wall filters to filter out generating primaries f1 and f2 so cubic distortion tone 2f1-f2 can be heard.

cy region. Listening to the amplified output of an ER-10C microphone placed in the ear would allow detection of tones at roughly 0 dB SPL; such tones would be just at the masked threshold produced by the amplified internal noise of the microphone. Otoacoustic emission tones at 5 to 15 dB SPL should be sufficiently above masked threshold to be both audible and tonal.

The only remaining problem is the presence of the primary tones. To filter out the primaries, we used two "brick wall filters" in series, each set to 1400 Hz as shown in Figure 8–5. Without the filter, the 65 and 55 dB SPL primary tones would mask the weak distortion tone we want to hear.

Figure 8–6 shows the section of Bach Partita #3 used for our demonstration recording. I am grateful to Dr. David Preves for suggesting this passage, whose rapidly alternating notes suggest two violins, and which uses notes that we could evoke in Tim's ear. (His ear doesn't play some notes as well as others, as you will hear when we play the demonstration tape.)

First I will play an old recording of the passage of music shown in Figure 8–6, so you have some idea of what you will be listening for when it is played by ear. (PLAYS: Band 4 on the enclosed CD.)

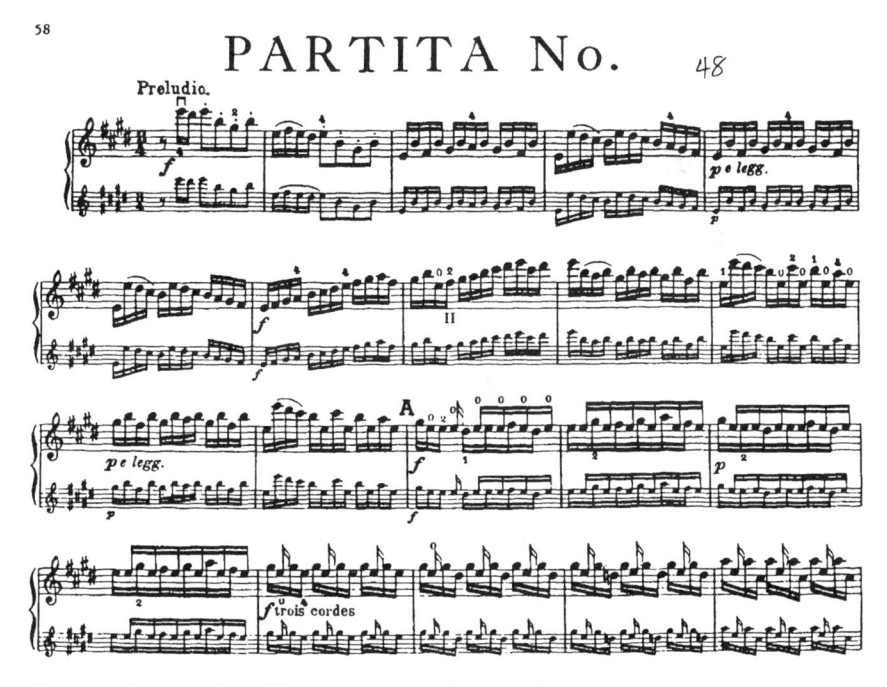

Figure 8–6. A portion of Bach Partita No. 3 played by ear.

The section starting at the bar marked "A" is the section that you will now hear as a recording of the cubic distortion tones produced in Tim's earcanal. We used computer control of the f2 oscillator to produce the frequencies shown in Table 8–1. Table 8–1 also shows the resultant cubic

TABLE 8–1. Frequencies used for generating the first two bars of the Bach Partita #3 demonstration, with primary f1 = Bb = 1864 Hz. All succeeding bars were generated in a like manner to those shown here.

CDT NOTE NUMBER	CDT NOTE NAME	CDT TONE FREQUENCY	f2 TONE FREQUENCY
1	G	1567	2161
2	Eb	1244	2484
3	Eb	1258	2470
4	Eb	1244	2484
5	D	1174	2554
6	Eb	1244	2484
7	Eb	1258	2470
8	Eb	1244	2484
9	F	1396	2332
10	Eb	1244	2484
11	D	1174	2554
12	Eb	1244	2484
13	Eb	1258	2470
14	Eb	1244	2484
15	G	1567	2161
16	Eb	1244	2484
17	F	1396	2332
18	Eb	1244	2484
19	G	1567	2161
20	Eb	1244	2484
21	A	1660	2068
22	Eb	1244	2484
23	F	1396	2332
24	Eb	1244	2484

Notes: 1. In an attempt to add realism, a small difference in frequency (10 cents or 10% of a semitone) was added between "downstroke of the bow" (e.g., note 3) and "upstroke of the bow" (note 4). The effect was hard to hear, probably not worth the bother, and slightly confuses the appearance of Table 8–1. 2. A subsequent calculation generated "vibrato," as described in the text. This *was* audible and improved the musicality of Tim's performance. 3. The Partita was transposed down a half-note for this recording.

distortion tone. Only the first two bars of music are displayed in Table 8–1. For naturalness, a small amount of vibrato was added to each note, changing f2 successively by 0, +20, 0, and −20 musical cents from the value shown (20 cents = 1.2%). (PLAYS: Band 5 on CD.) We later made recordings at half these frequencies (this one was an octave above the written part), which were also successful (Plays: Band 6 on CD).

Any musician in the audience with perfect pitch is perhaps wondering why we had the ear play the passage 1/2 note flat. I confess I can't remember why I transposed the passage down a 1/2 note on the computer before generating the f2 file, although it seemed to make sense at the time.

The experimentalists in the audience are probably asking how we know that the tones we hear came from Tim's ear rather than being generated by some form of intermodulation distortion in the equipment.

The question can be answered by making a recording in an ear which presents the proper acoustic impedance but generates no emissions; that is, a dead ear. An ideal dead ear is the Zwislocki Coupler. The next recording was made identically to the last, except that the probe was removed from Tim's ear and placed in Zwislocki's coupler. Since Tim's ear has a measured acoustic impedance close to that of the Zwislocki coupler, any equipment distortion should show up as tones in the "dead ear." This distortion problem occasionally plagues some commercial otoacoustic emission measurement equipment; the test is the same. (PLAYS: Band 7 on CD. I trust you did not hear Bach playing this time. There is a small bleed-through Bb tone, which is the f1 primary, but no melody.)

A REVIEW OF HEARING, WITH THE GOAL OF DESCRIBING THREE TYPES OF HEARING LOSS

Distortion Products as Indication of Outer Hair Cell Function

We have already had quite a bit of discussion about the operation of the outer hair cells, but the next two figures may be interesting nonetheless. Figure 8–7 shows the different distortion products generated in a normal ear by the nonlinearity of the outer hair cell motion. These were measured using the CUB^{e}DIS™ system. Note that the harmonic-distortion products are evident at 2f1 and 2f2, as is the difference tone at f2-f1. Both third-order distortion tones are visible: the Tartini tone is the lower cubic distortion tone (CDT) at 2f1-f2. The upper CDT is at 2f2-f1. The 2f1-f2 tone is the one we measure clinically to generate the "DP-gram."

Figure 8–8 contains data that I find particularly interesting. It shows the DP-gram and audiogram of a 35 year old female Swedish musician who is also a television producer. When she visited our laboratory, she

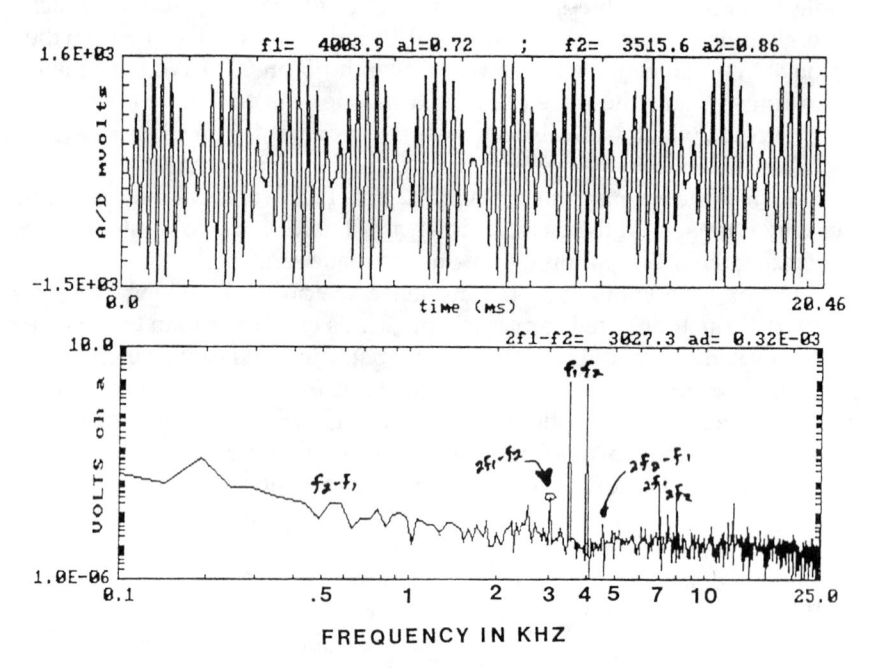

Figure 8–7. Spectrogram of distortion products from the ear: Waveform of combined 65-dB SPL primary tones shown in top graph, spectrum analysis of earcanal microphone output shown in bottom graph.

confessed she produced a lot of rock music and she thought she had a small noise-induced notch in her audiogram. When I measured her otoacoustic emissions, we saw that her emissions were 20–30 dB above the noise floor until we got to 6 kHz, where they dropped not quite to the noise floor and then returned to normal at 8 kHz. I measured her threshold audiogram with the result you see: normal hearing through 4 kHz, a dip at 6 kHz, and normal at 8 kHz. (Before you buy otoacoustic-emission equipment to measure audiograms, I should confess that Figure 8–8 represents the nicest correlation between audiogram and DP-gram that I have seen. By the time most such subjects come in for testing, they have a 50–60 dB hearing loss at the notch frequency, and appreciable loss at adjacent audiometric frequencies.)

For our present purposes, the interesting question is: "What happens to loudness growth as outer hair cell (and inner hair cell) function is lost?"

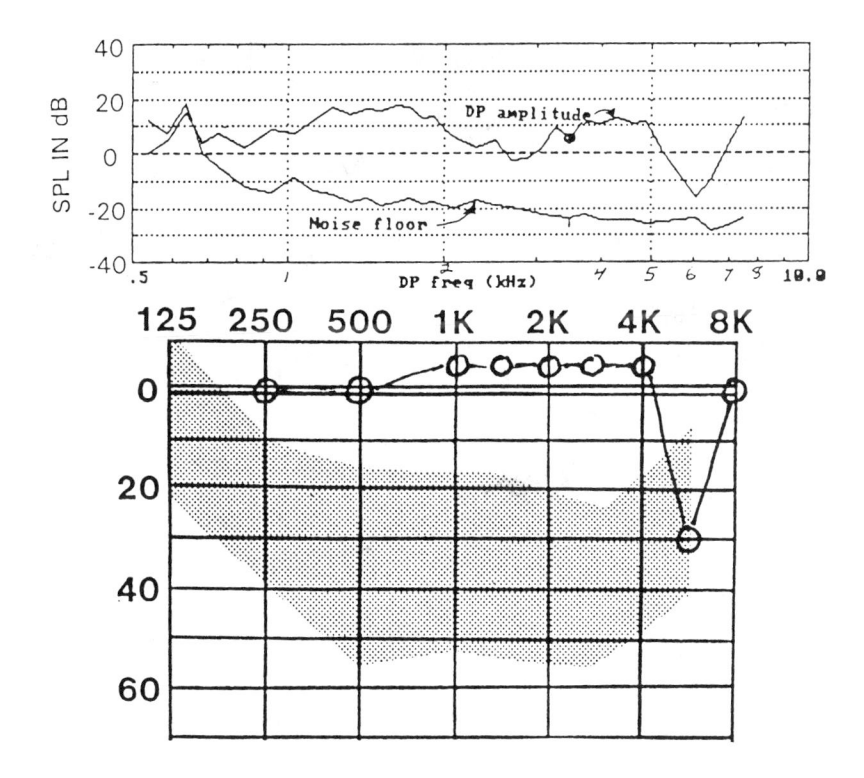

DPE AND PURE-TONE AUDIOGRAM OF 35 YEAR OLD FEMALE WHO "PRODUCED AND RECORDED ROCK MUSIC"

Figure 8-8. DP-gram and audiogram of 35 year old woman with apparent loss of outer hair cell function only near 6 kHz.

The Operation of the Cochlea According to Berlin

First, I'd like to give a demonstration of the operation of the cochlea, a demonstration I learned from Dr. Berlin and have used in nearly every lecture since then.

Figure 8-9 shows a drawing of the cochlea with outer hair cells, inner hair cells, neurons, and the tectorial membrane. The drawing shows the outer hair cells embedded in the tectorial membrane and the inner hair cells as nearly or just touching the tectorial membrane.

From thousands of 8th nerve recordings, we know that all the signals going to the brain come from the inner hair cells. So what do the outer

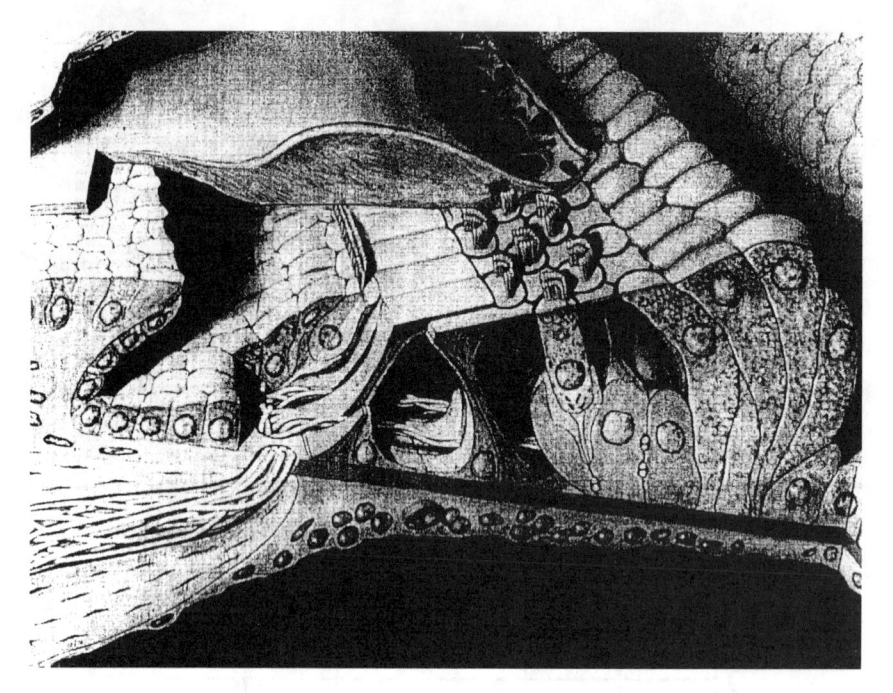

Figure 8–9. Drawing of cochlea showing inner and outer hair cells, neurons, and tectorial membrane.

hair cells do? Let us assume Dr. Berlin's arm is the tectorial membrane, and my fingers intertwined with his fingers represent the embedded outer hair cell fibers. There are various hypotheses on the exact mechanism by which the inner hair cells are induced to fire, and on how the outer hair cells increase the sensitivity of the cochlea by 40 dB or more. My personal favorite is that the motion of the outer hair cells modulates the gap between the tectorial membrane and the stereocilia of the inner hair cells. Because the fluid flow resistance varies as the third power of the gap spacing, only a small motion would produce the required 40 dB change in sensitivity: changing the gap from 10 microns down to 2 microns would do the trick, for example. For our present purposes, however, we are going to assume that the inner hair cells—represented by the fingers of my free hand—fire when they bump into the tectorial membrane, represented by the underside of Dr. Berlin's arm above the elbow. For this simulation, I am holding my fingers in the rest position about 2 inches away. With no help from the outer hair cells, the inner hair cells will fire when a 40 or 50 dB SPL input causes enough motion to bridge that 2-inch gap so the inner hair cell fibers bump against the tectorial membrane, as the fingers of my free hand in motion bump against my assistant's upper arm.

With the assumed mechanical amplification correlated with normal outer hair cell motion, however, only about 10 dB SPL is required in order to produce the required amount of motion between the inner hair cell stereocilia and the tectorial membrane. With the help of the outer hair cell amplifiers, firing occurs with only 10 dB SPL or so (roughly 0 dB HL) at the eardrum.

If the outer hair cells are damaged or missing or paralyzed, it will take something like 50 dB SPL (40 dB HL) to cause the inner hair cells to fire. In other words, we will see a 40 dB hearing loss.

What happens to loud sounds with this model? Let us consider a 90-dB SPL input. If 50 dB causes 2 inches of motion in our simulation, then 90-dB SPL would cause 200 inches of motion: the required motion of my free hand would extend down 16 feet from where it is to somewhere in the basement below us. With 200 inches of motion available, the 2 inches of motion available from the outer hair cell amplifiers becomes irrelevant. With such a large motion available, the inner hair cells will fire whether the outer hair cells move or not. We conclude that with high-intensity signals the inner hair cells should fire normally.

The remaining question is: "How can one experience more than a 40- or 50-dB cochlear hearing *loss* if the outer hair cell amplifiers only provide 40–50 dB of *gain*?" The answer is that the same aural abuse—from shooting, using a chain saw, or whatever you did that broke off the hairs of your outer hair cells—the same abuse that broke off your outer hair cells will sooner or later be likely to break off the stereocilia of the inner hair cells as well. Loss of inner hair cells results not only in a loss of sensitivity, but a loss of "channel capacity" in the auditory system: Fewer transmitting sites are available to send information to the brain. (It is also possible for the tectorial membrane to float up and away—I think I first heard this suggestion from Dr. Berlin—causing a loss of firing sensitivity for the inner hair cells at high levels even though the inner hair cells themselves may be undamaged.) In most cases, however, histological evidence suggests that the mechanism for hearing loss above 40–50 dB HL is a loss of inner hair cells and the consequent loss of auditory channel capacity.

LOUDNESS GROWTH DATA

Most of the early loudness-growth data were obtained at Bell Telephone Laboratories. Those earlier data look much like the more recent data of Lyregaard (1988) and Lippman et al. (1977), shown idealized in Figure 8–10.

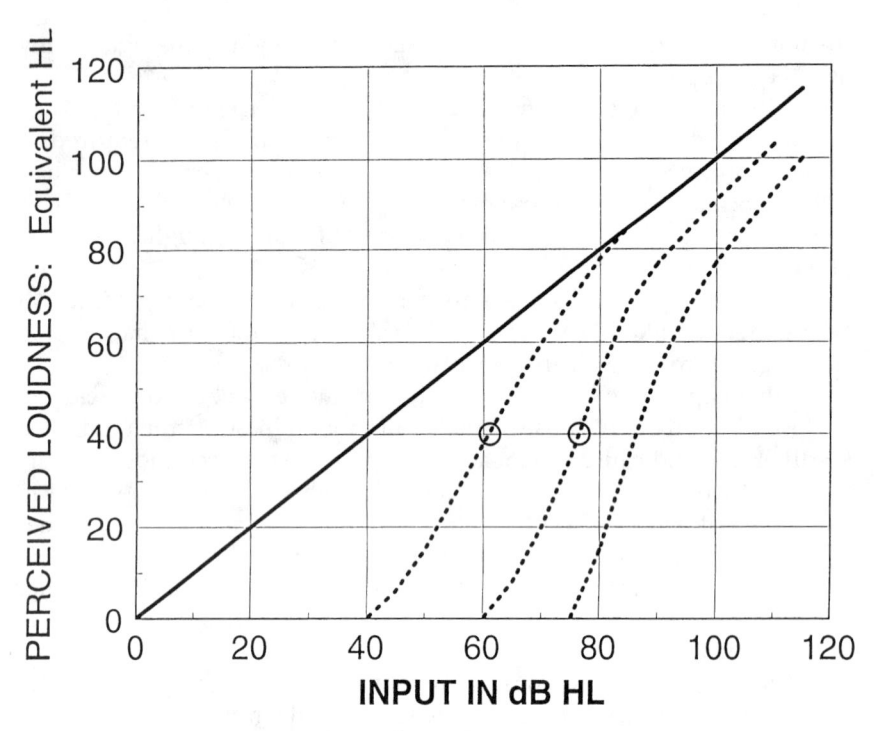

Figure 8–10. Idealized normal and impaired loudness growth curves for 40, 60, and 75 dB hearing loss, after data of Lyregaard (1988) and Lippman (1977).

Note that somewhat like using the early phon scale from Bell Labs, Lyregaard choose to plot loudness not in terms of judged magnitude (as is often done in psychoacoustics), but in terms of equivalent loudness for subjects who hear normally. I like this simplification: If the average subject with normal hearing judges a tone presented at 40 dB hearing level as having a loudness magnitude of 2.3 on the Pascoe/Hawkins scale (2 = soft, 3 = comfortable but soft), the corresponding point is plotted as 40 dB HL on the Y axis, not 2.3. If someone with a hearing impairment requires a 61 dB HL tone in order to have a loudness experience of magnitude 2.3, you plot that point in the same manner, as 40 dB HL on the Y axis above 65 dB on the X-axis. If another individual requires 76 dB HL for the same loudness judgment of 2.3, this is plotted as the x,y point (76,40). (These examples correspond to the circled points on Figure 8–10).

The are two other important sets of recent loudness data to consider. Figure 8–11 shows the data of Pascoe (1988), who reported on 500 ears tested at 0.5, 1, 2, and 4 kHz. Finding nearly the same curves applied at all frequencies, he combined data across frequency. By taking the normal

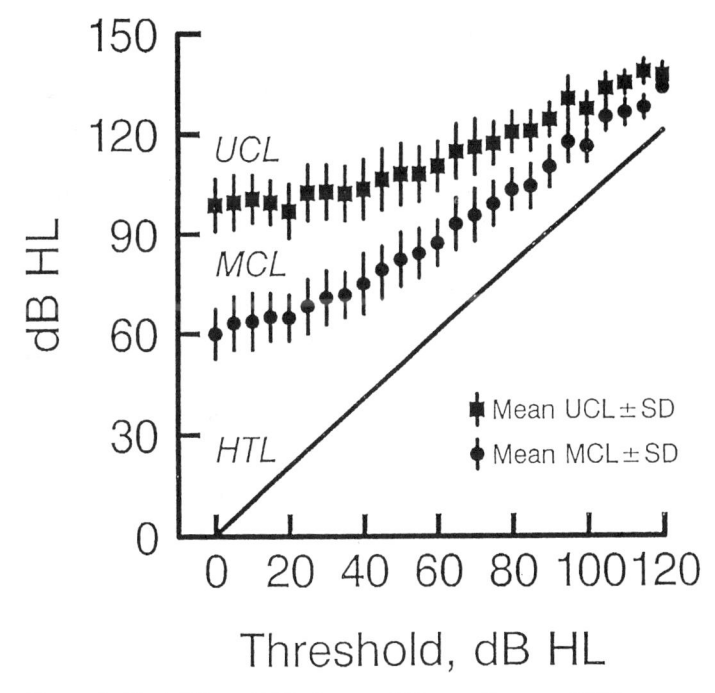

Figure 8–11. MCL and LDL data on 508 ears (Pascoe, 1988).

LDL (Loudness Discomfort Level) as reference, and noting the amount of elevation above normal LDL accompanying a given degree of hearing loss, we can obtain an estimate of whether or not a given amount of gain for loud sounds is likely to cause discomfort. More precisely, it provides an estimate of the *amount* of gain for high-level sounds that can be safely provided if the average individual with impaired hearing is to be no more at risk of loudness discomfort than a neighbor with normal hearing sitting nearby. This is an extraordinarily important piece of information that we will use later.

The other recent data are those of Hellman and Meiselman (1993). Hellman and her colleagues have been doing a variety of loudness studies using cross-modality loudness matching, direct loudness magnitude estimation, and loudness production (where the subject chooses the signal level that matches an assigned loudness magnitude target). Pleasantly enough, they obtained basically the same answer with each approach. Even more importantly, they have studied a large number of subjects with hearing loss: 17 people with 45 dB loss, 24 with 55 dB loss, 20 with 65 dB loss, and 20 with 75 dB loss. (Each loss category included losses within 5 dB of the nominal value.)

Figure 8–12 shows the Hellman and Meiselman data plotted as Lyregaard had done. (A note of thanks: At the time I became aware of the Hellman and Meiselman data, I had already extracted curves from the Lyregaard and Lippman et al. data. Dr. Hellman was kind enough to transform her data to a form ready for the plot of Figure 8–12.) Figure 8–13 shows a comparison between the Hellman and Meiselman data and the previous estimate for a typical subject with 40-dB loss. Her data, taken on a large number of subjects, look quite similar to the earlier estimate based on the Lyregaard and Lippman data. Figure 8–14 shows a similar comparison for 60-dB loss. Again, the estimated 60-dB curve is largely bracketed by the Hellman and Meiselman data for 55- and 65-dB losses.[3]

---

[3]The recent high-level data are sometimes sparse because of Institutional Review Boards, even though there is sometimes little logical reason for the limitations that are set. For example, 100 dB HL is, depending on the frequency, about 105 dB SPL in the sound field, no big deal for a short exposure. Country and western bands sometimes produce 100–105 dB SPL for hours at audiology meetings! During routine practice, an amateur violinist (the writer, for example) can produce 106 dB SPL at the external ear for a short period of time. A virtuoso can produce over 112 dB, 4 times the power, *and* a beautiful tone! The use of short-duration signals of 110 dB SPL and higher is needed in order to obtain clear-cut LDL measurements in order to facilitate hearing aid design research.

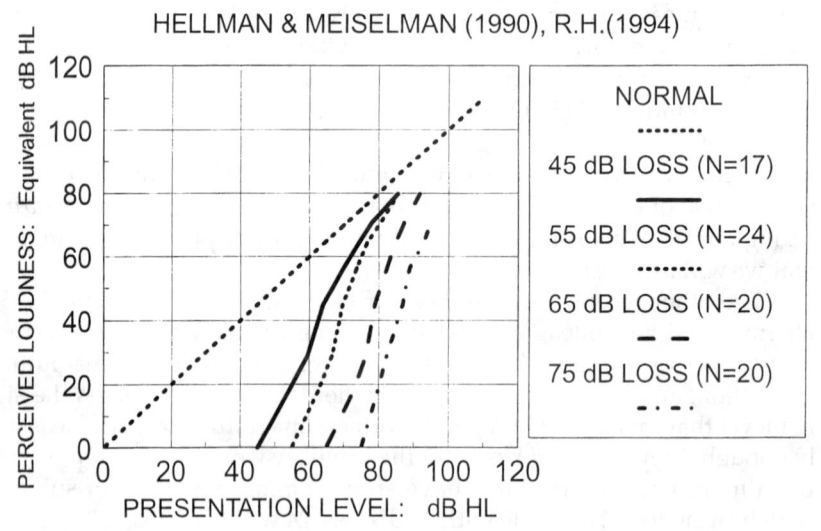

Figure 8–12. Loudness from cross-modality matching.

LOUDNESS GROWTH: TYPE I LOSS (40 dB)

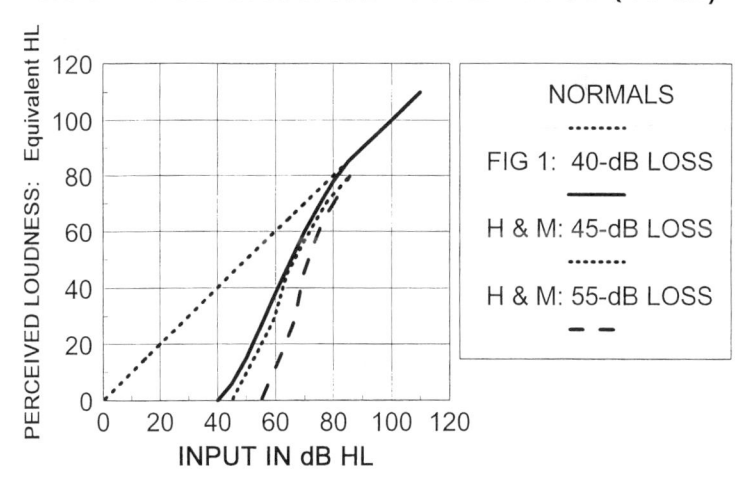

NORMALS ········
FIG 1: 40-dB LOSS ——
H & M: 45-dB LOSS ········
H & M: 55-dB LOSS – –

Figure 8–13. Killion & Fikret-Pasa comparison of the earlier loudness-growth estimate for a 40 dB loss with the Hellman & Meiselman data for 45 and 55 dB losses.

LOUDNESS GROWTH: TYPE II LOSS (60 dB)

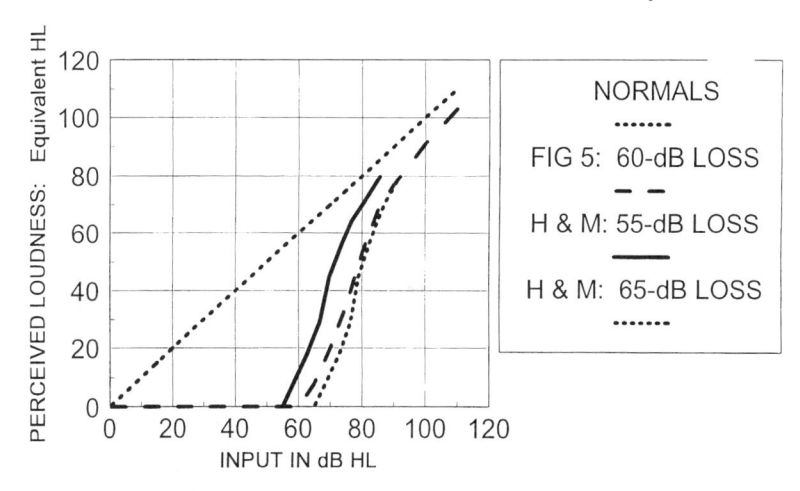

NORMALS ········
FIG 5: 60-dB LOSS – –
H & M: 55-dB LOSS ——
H & M: 65-dB LOSS ········

Figure 8–14. Killion & Fikret-Pasa comparison of the earlier loudness-growth estimate for a 60 dB loss with the Hellman & Meiselman data for 55 and 65 dB losses.

We now have everything in place to talk about types of hearing loss, and the types of hearing aid processing they might require.

Types of Hearing Loss

Figure 8–15 illustrates three types of hearing loss (Killion & Fikret-Pasa, 1993). A fourth type—profound loss—is not shown because we know less about it.

Type I hearing loss is depicted in the upper left panel of Figure 8–15, where the loudness growth for a typical cochlear loss of 40 dB is illustrat-

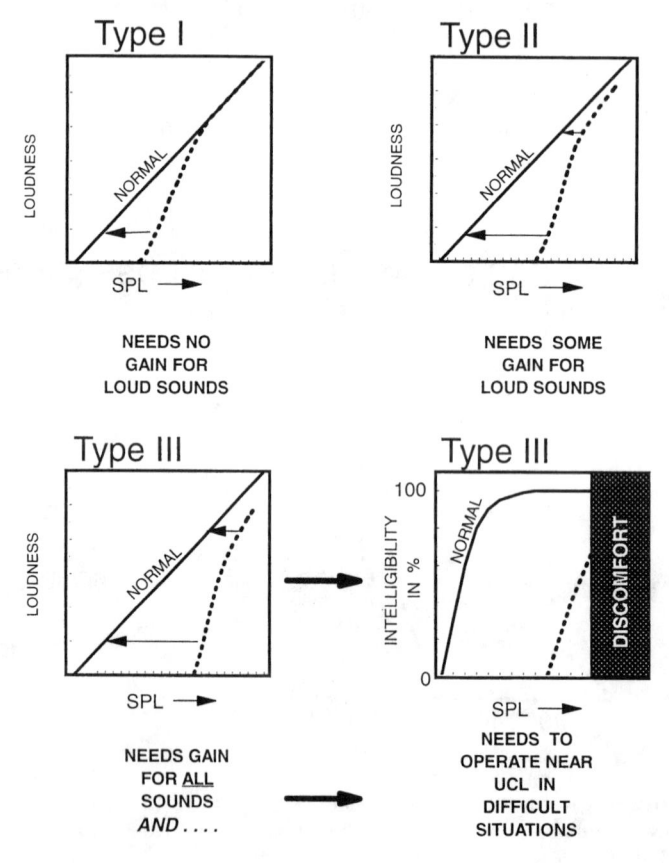

Figure 8–15. The three types of hearing loss.

ed. A Type I loss shows complete recruitment: loudness sensation for intense sounds is the same as normal, but sounds below 40-dB HL are inaudible. This finding is consistent with a loss of outer hair cell function with normal inner hair cell function. With increasing level above 40 dB HL, loudness gradually returns to normal. Not only has *loudness* returned to normal for high-level sounds, but you can find subjects with 40-dB threshold loss who appear to have normal or near-normal high-level hearing by *any* measure you apply. This is true whether you measure high-level difference limens for intensity or frequency, psychoacoustic tuning curves, electrical auditory brainstem response (ABR), or speech discrimination in noise. In animals, where it is possible to place an electrode in the 8th nerve bundle, individual neural recordings can be normal at high levels in the region of loss. Many of these findings were reviewed 15 years ago (Killion, 1979).

To repeat: An individual with Type I hearing loss has a *loss of sensitivity for quiet sounds*, but may have little or no loss of hearing for loud sounds. The hearing loss is restricted to low-level sounds. Although we will discuss hearing aids in greater detail later, it already seems evident that *an individual with a Type I loss doesn't need loud sounds to be made any louder than they already are*; what is needed is gain for low-level sounds in order to make them audible and clear. Not so evident—as witnessed by some hearing aid designs—is the conclusion that the individual with a Type I hearing loss doesn't need loud sounds to be made any *quieter* than they are. In other words, no output *limiting* for loud sounds is needed, at least not unless people with normal hearing also need hearing protection in the same environment. A corollary of this conclusion is that is a mistake to choose a low maximum output "SSPL-90" for a Type I loss; it will only result in premature clipping and distortion of everyday loud sounds. This conclusion is consistent with the experimental findings of Fortune, Preves, and Woodruff (1991), who reported fewer complaints of discomfort with the Class D hearing aids, which had the *highest* undistorted output.

A Type II hearing loss is shown in the upper right panel of Figure 8–15, where the loudness growth for a Type II loss of 60 dB is illustrated. A loss of 60 dB is probably too great to explain solely on the basis of a loss of outer hair cell function, and requires that we assume some inner hair cell loss as well. With a Type II loss, we thus have not only a loss of sensitivity for quiet sounds, but also a loss of some speech cues as well. A loss of inner hair cells means there is less information available to be transmitted to the brain, even for intense sounds. So not only is more gain required for low-level sounds with a Type II loss, but some gain will be required to restore even *loud* sounds to normal loudness.

The loss of inner hair cells means, however, that even with the 8 or 10 dB of gain required to make intense sounds normally loud (see Figures 8–14 & 8–15), there will usually still be a deficit in intelligibility for speech, especially in noise; fewer of the redundant speech cues will be available to the brain's processing centers. It is the availability of redundant speech cues that gives persons with normal hearing their remarkable resistance to interference from noise (Villchur, 1993). Persons with normal hearing can listen simultaneously to four talkers, for example, and selectively choose which conversation to follow. Individuals with a Type II (or worse) loss typically have a reduced ability to do that even with the best of hearing aid fittings (although they can do dramatically better than with the traditional hearing aid fittings of yesterday).

A Type III loss is shown in the lower panels of Figure 8–15, where both the loudness growth and the *intelligibility* function for a Type III loss of perhaps 75 dB are shown. When the hearing loss has progressed into the 70 to 80 dB region, loudness ceases to be a primary concern; the inner hair cell loss (and the resultant loss of normally redundant speech cues) is so great that one concern dominates: intelligibility. Moreover, the range of input SPLs over which speech is intelligible—especially when noise is present—is often very narrow. We no longer have the luxury of a large range of levels over which speech can be understood in noise.

Data for one subject with Type III hearing loss are shown in Figure 8–16. This subject was the first of eight Type-III-loss subjects studied by Fikret-Pasa (1993). This subject obtained a word recognition score of 60% in four-talker babble noise when the test was presented at a level just below discomfort. With a 5 dB reduction in level, the score dropped 10%; with a 10 dB reduction the intelligibility had dropped to half. The useful dynamic range of this subject in difficult listening situations is 5–10 dB on the HL dial.

Hearing-Aid Input-Output Desiderata

It is clear that a Type III hearing loss requires a totally different hearing aid than the first two. In a difficult listening situation, the only chance for someone with a Type III hearing loss to understand speech is to have everything presented at close to discomfort level.[4] At a party, for example, such an individual needs a hearing aid that allows sufficient gain to

---

[4] I am indebted to Harry Teder, one of Fikret-Pasa's subjects, for first bringing this phenomenon to my understanding. He observed that an experimental Adaptive-Compression® limiting hearing aid, similar to the one he normally used but with a 5 dB reduction in output, was inadequate for his loss. With that reduced output, he found himself handicapped at a party, migrating toward the quieter fringes because of greatly increased difficulty in carrying on a conversation in noise. Type III loss might well be called "Teder loss," since he first clearly understood and described the phenomenon.

INTELLIGIBILITY VS. SPL FOR SUBJECT

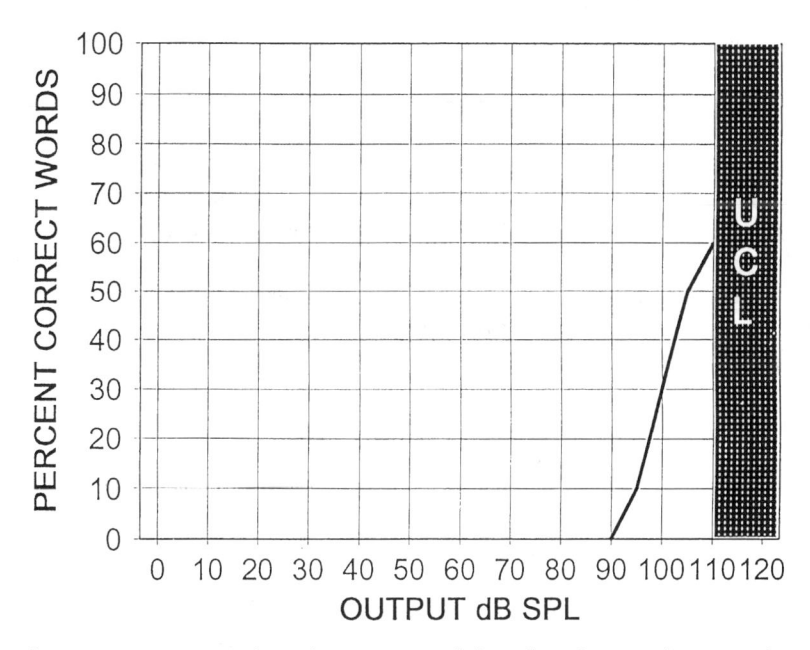

Figure 8–16. Measured word recognition ability of a subject with Type III hearing loss (Subject 1 from 1989 Fikret-Pasa study).

bring all of the ebb and flow of conversation to *beyond* discomfort, accompanied by appropriate compression limiting to keep all sounds just *below* discomfort. With this approach, all sounds will automatically be brought to the level of maximum intelligibility below discomfort. The only alternatives for an individual with a Type III loss are repeated volume control adjustment, regular discomfort, or loss of communication.

With Type I and Type II losses, on the other hand, restoration of normal loudness experience is a reasonable first goal. It is clearly the sensible goal in the case of a Type I loss. The argument goes as follows: Given (a) the need for sufficient gain to make quiet sounds audible and (b) the lack of need for any gain for high-level sounds, what is the most logical choice of gain for levels in-between?

The question can be answered by a reference to music. Assuming that the enjoyment of music is nearly universally desired, the existence of a loudness scale that has been in use in musical scores for more than 200 years would suggest that restoration of normal loudness experience would be a desirable thing in and of itself. The musical loudness scale ranges from ppp (extremely soft) through pp, p, mp, mf, f, and ff to fff (extremely loud),[5] not unlike recent 7-point loudness scales recommended by Pascoe (1988), Hawkins, Walden, Montgomery, and Prosek (1987), and the others.

What should we do about discomfort? The 102–106 dB SPL fff produced by the Chicago Symphony Orchestra at a 1st balcony seat would be uncomfortably loud for those with normal hearing if it lasted for more than a few seconds at a time. This observation suggests that normal musical enjoyment for individuals with Type I hearing loss would probably *not* be enhanced by arbitrary output limiting circuits to prevent discomfort, especially of the peak-detecting variety. Such circuits would detract from musical enjoyment by limiting the excitement of a great performance. (That has been my personal hearing-aid listening-test experience.) As argued below, such individuals don't need such protection unless they are forced to endure gain for loud sounds.

The argument for loudness restoration in the case of a Type II loss is not quite so self evident, although it appears to be the most sensible answer to the question "What should the hearing aid do at levels between quiet—where some 40 dB of gain is required—and intense—where only 8–10 dB is required to restore loudness?" Certainly *failing* to attempt some loudness restoration leads back to traditional linear hearing aids and the frequent volume-control adjustments they require. ("I have to adjust my volume controls *all* the time during a church service," complained one wearer of good Class D linear hearing aids.)

If we assume for the moment that restoration of normal loudness is the first order of business, then it readily follows from the curves in Figures 8–13 to 8–16 that the gain of the hearing aid should decrease gradually as the input level increases. This is exactly what wide dynamic range compression accomplishes, and it is the *only* compression or automatic-gain-control (AGC) system that does so.

Again note that the goal suitable for Type I and Type II loss—loudness restoration—is in sharp contrast to the goal for Type III loss. What is needed with Type III loss is a high-gain linear hearing aid with output *limiting*, preferably using variable-release-time compression, with the

---

[5] I have recently seen a marking of ffff for the final chord of a church-choir anthem—the composer presumably trying to exhort the choristers to some kind of superhuman effort—but a 7- or 8-point loudness scale appears adequate for most musical and clinical purposes. Some forms of rock music provide a possible exception. A VU meter hardly wiggles while monitoring some rock-music broadcasts, indicating a 2-point loudness scale might be adequate.

limiting set just below discomfort.[6] With the volume control turned up, everything is brought *near* discomfort to maximize intelligibility, but *below* discomfort to avoid discomfort.

Figure 8–17 shows that available wide-dynamic-range-compression (WDRC) hearing aid circuits can provide nearly perfect loudness compensation for a typical Type I hearing loss. Note that no gain *or loss* is provided for high-level inputs, consistent with the normal or near-normal high-level hearing with Type I losses.

TYPE I HEARING LOSS WITH WDRC PROCESSING

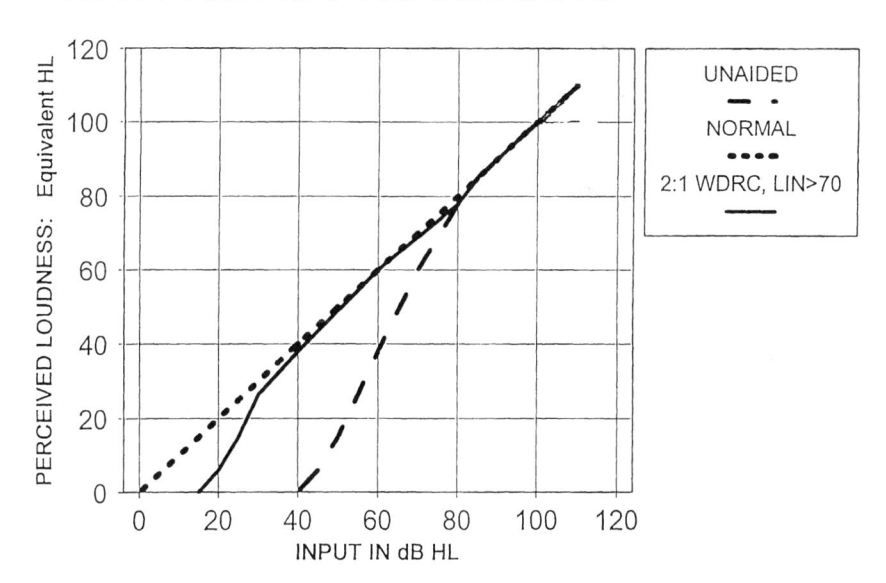

Figure 8–17. Restoration of loudness for a 40 dB Type I hearing loss using a commercial wide-dynamic-range-compression hearing aid amplifier. Note: The full fortissississimo (fff) output of the Chicago Symphony Orchestra does not cause clipping.

---

[6]The data of Fikret-Pasa (1993) indicate variable-release-time compression limiting can provide some individuals with Type III hearing loss an improvement of 5 dB or more in effective signal-to-noise ratio, compared to conventional compression limiting with 50 mS recovery time, when both are driven deep into limiting.

Physiological Data and WDRC Hearing Aids

Dr. Brownell was kind enough to lend me one of the slides he used during his talk, a slide of the Ruggero and Rich (1990) data relating measured basilar-membrane velocity to input SPL. That slide is shown here replotted as curve B.M.#L14 in Figure 8–18. As described earlier, a large gain is seen for low-level inputs, a gain which disappears for high-level inputs. When the outer hair cells are paralyzed with furosemide so they can't move, the gain disappears at all levels, giving evidence that the gain is provided by the action of the outer hair cells themselves.

Since the time of my verbal presentation, I have been unable to resist generating the comparison shown in Table 8–2 between the action of the outer hair cell amplifiers in the cochlea, using the B.M.#13 curve in Figure 8–18, and the action of a popular hearing aid amplifier which uses wide-dynamic-range compression (WDRC). The compression ratio for the ear was derived by first converting velocity to dB. The compression ratio was then calculated as (dB change in input)/(dB change in output). Note: In Figure 3 of the same paper, Ruggero & Rich (1991) reported what they

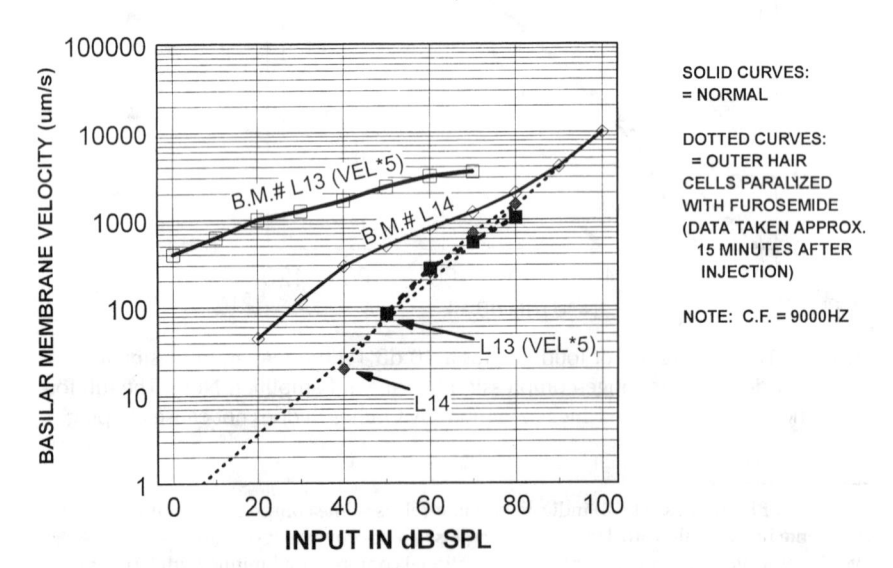

Figure 8–18. Ruggero and Rich (1991) data on the operation of Corti's organ as a wide-dynamic-range-compression amplifier.

TABLE 8–2.

AMPLIFIER TYPE:	Outer Hair Cell Amplifier (Sample #14, 9 kHz C.F.)	Wide-Dynamic-Range Compression Amplifier (4 kHz test frequency)
LOWER THRESHOLD OF COMPRESSION	35 dB	40 dB
UPPER THRESHOLD OF COMPRESSION	85 dB	90 dB
COMPRESSION RATIO	2.3:1	2.1:1
GAIN INCREASE FOR QUIET SOUNDS	20-50 dB	25 dB
POWER CONSUMPTION	50 uWatts	230 uWatts

consider to be a better measurement on another animal, data that can be extrapolated to indicate 50 dB of gain at 10 dB SPL, and little or no gain at 90 dB SPL. Those data (B.M.#L13) have been normalized and added to Figure 8–18.

It is clear from Table 8–2 that nature provides a substantial battery economy: Some 15,000 outer hair cell amplifiers operate on less than 50 uWatts total;[7] a single WDRC hearing aid amplifier requires 230 uWatts.

It is also clear from Figure 8–18 that nature does not normally provide us with linear hearing, but hearing which provides increased sensitivity for quiet sounds and a gradual reduction of sensitivity with increasing level. Thus, nature normally provides wide dynamic range compression to increase gain for low-level sounds! The only time the human ear shows a linear input-output function is when the outer hair cells are missing or temporarily paralyzed. Either causes a 40–50 dB hearing loss. Linear amplification is "pathological."

---

[7]The power consumption of the cochlea was estimated two ways. First, the vascularization of the cochlea was extracted as a list of diameters by microscopic examination of a temporal bone slide. The sum of the inverse fourth power of those diameters gave a total relative flow, which was compared to the inverse fourth power of the diameter (1 cm) of the aorta. This gave a presumed power ratio of 70:10^9. Considering the short-term 1 horsepower (745 watt) maximum output of a human, this implies approximately a 50 uWatt supply to the cochlea. A similar figure was derived from the measured resistivity/mm of the cochlear fluid and the 80 mV battery supported by the stria vascularis. The two estimates were within a factor of two of each other, indicating that 50 uWatts is probably a good figure.

Wide Dynamic Range Compression (WDRC) Amplifiers

Figure 8–19 shows a presumed ideal input-output characteristic suitable for a hearing aid, inferred 16 years ago from available loudness-growth data for sensorineural hearing loss (Killion, 1979). This graph shows substantial gain for quiet sounds, gradually decreasing as input SPL increases, until no gain (or loss) is provided for loud sounds. A similar ideal characteristic was suggested by Barford (1978). The striking similarity to the physiological input-output curve shown in Figure 8–18, added to this figure as the dotted curve, is evident. The input-output function of the commercial WDRC amplifier looks very much like the normal nonlinear input-output function of the cochlea.

It might seem surprising that an electronic amplifier—designed in the 1970s before the recent physiological data became available—should match the ear's physiological amplifier so well. Recall, however, that psychoacoustic data on the input-output characteristic of normal-hearing and impaired ears have been available since the 1930s. The physiological data have simply supplied a reassuring explanation for what we already believed to be true.

Indeed, Steinberg and Gardner (1937) first concluded from loudness data on impaired ears that what we now call wide-dynamic-range com-

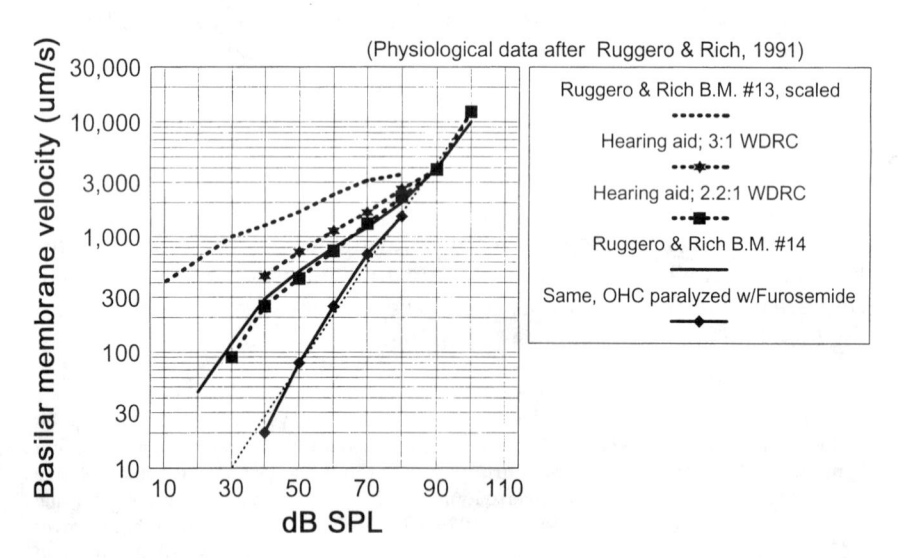

Figure 8–19. Presumed ideal characteristic for hearing aid amplifier (Killion, 1978), compared to physiological input-output function measured by Ruggero and Rich (1991).

pression[8] was required in a hearing aid amplifier: "Owing to the expanding action of this type of loss it would be necessary to introduce a corresponding compression in the amplifier in order to produce the same amplification at all levels" (p. 20). Ironically, it took nearly 30 years before Goldberg (1966) introduced wearable low-distortion WDRC hearing aid amplifiers into the marketplace. I can recall listening to one of his BTE "Computer" hearing aids in 1968, and marveling that his factory-programmable-compression-ratio amplifier was not used in every hearing aid. (Goldberg's amplifiers still sound good.)

Only in this decade, however, have WDRC amplifiers become widely accepted; over 50 years after Steinberg and Gardner's observations. Today several commercial hearing aid amplifiers in addition to Goldberg's can produce excellent compensation for the pathological loudness growth of sensorineural loss. The hearing aid design based on Villchur's research (1973) allows choice of compression ratio (Waldhauer & Villchur, 1988); another design (Killion, 1979) has trimpot control (soon to be computer-programmable control) of compression ratio.

Figure 8–20 shows that not all "compression" hearing aids can be set to compensate for the impaired loudness function. The irony is that the one which fails most visibly has often been described in lectures as having the capability of being programmable to be "just like" a popular WDRC amplifier with treble-increases-at-low-level (TILL) operation. The thin solid curve shown in Figure 8–20 was plotted from the manufacturer's published data. This circuit is a substantial improvement over linear hearing aids, and does a good job of loudness compensation up to about 70-dB SPL input, but the 40 dB range of normally loud and very loud sounds is suppressed. This aid is *not* just like a good WDRC-TILL hearing aid, which preserves normal loudness experience for *all* input levels! For all practical purposes, the aid programmed as shown in Figure 8–20 operates as a compression limiter above 70 dB. This should be a good aid for a Type III hearing loss, where its programmable limiting should be useful, but hardly ideal for Type I or Type II losses.

This argument deserves more discussion. The region between 70 and 110 dB is where most of the excitement in music resides. When the members of the orchestra are performing at physiological limits in order to produce the excitement of a Mahler finale, it will come out of the thin-solid-curve aid sounding a little like a tiny tinkle. The last 40 dB of excitement has been thrown away. It is analogous to saying "I want no more

---

[8]Wide-dynamic-range compression was what was meant by the word "compression" at Bell Labs in those days; what we now call compression limiting was simply called limiting. Limiting due to peak clipping was called peak clipping.

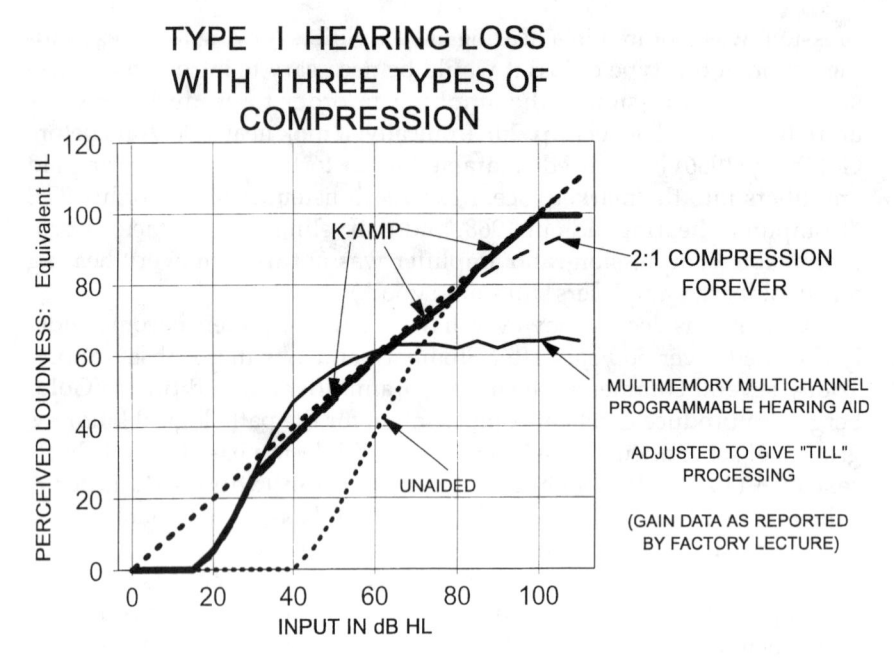

TYPE I HEARING LOSS WITH THREE TYPES OF COMPRESSION

(Figure: Perceived Loudness (Equivalent HL) vs. Input in dB HL, showing curves for K-AMP, 2:1 COMPRESSION FOREVER, MULTIMEMORY MULTICHANNEL PROGRAMMABLE HEARING AID ADJUSTED TO GIVE "TILL" PROCESSING (GAIN DATA AS REPORTED BY FACTORY LECTURE), and UNAIDED.)

Figure 8–20. Amplified loudness growth for several compression hearing aids.

than a 150 watt light bulb to illuminate my life. I am going to accept the range between moonlight and 150 watts, nothing above that. Never do I wish to see bright sunshine again." Even worse from the standpoint of naturalness would be the use of an AGC system that forced all sounds to the *same* loudness (the most comfortable loudness level has been suggested). That would be equivalent to eliminating the brightness both from 150 watts up to sunlight *and* from 150 watts down to moonlight.

The auditory equivalent of bright sunshine *can* be obtained with an output-limiting aid by turning up the volume control, but then most *everyday* sounds will be too loud, as illustrated in Figure 8–21, and a 40-dB wide range of sounds will be brought to just short of discomfort. Moreover, visual and auditory discomfort is a time-dependent phenomenon. I find that driving down the road on a sunny day is no problem for short periods of time, but after 5–10 minutes my eyes start to ache. Similarly, the 100–105 dB levels at a country and western dance are OK for a few minutes, but after that I get out my Musician's Earplugs. Levels that provide an exciting few seconds of finale to an orchestral performance become uncomfortable when prolonged into minutes. This means that sunglasses sufficiently dark for hours of light exposure, or output-limiting levels sufficiently low for hours of high-level sound exposure, may provide excessive attenuation for transient conditions.

Output limiting for Type I and Type II loss is so obviously wrong that we must ask ourselves how we arrived at the use of limiting (compression or peak clipping) for Type I and Type II losses in the first place. I believe it came about because the only amplification available over the years was linear amplification. With only linear amplification available, some form of limiting is absolutely necessary because unlimited amplification of high-level real-world sounds by the amount required for quiet sounds would cause pain or physiological damage. Such linear amplifiers inherently included limiting by peak clipping, which, chosen appropriately, would prevent discomfort. Low-distortion compression limiting was such an obvious and dramatic improvement over limiting by clipping (see, e.g., Hawkins & Naidoo, 1993, or Fikret-Pasa, 1993) that we

TYPE I HEARING LOSS WITH LINEAR PROCESSING

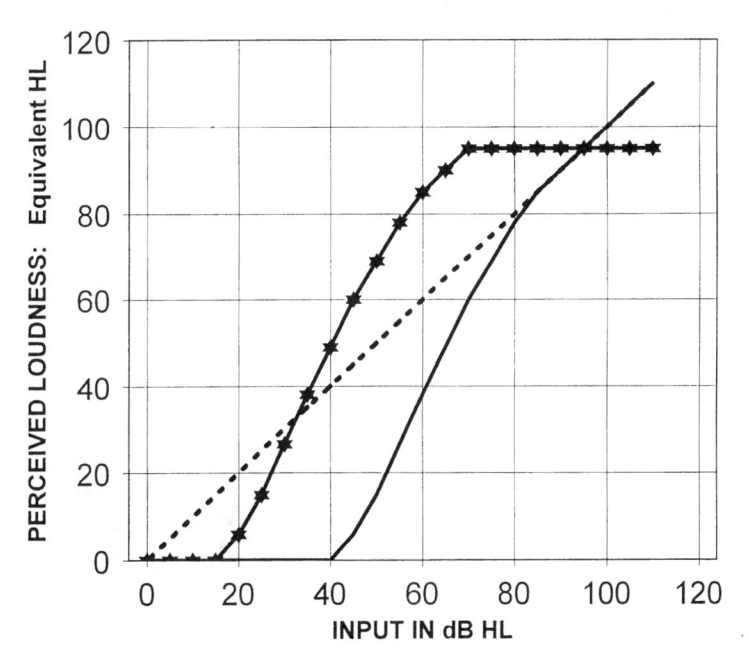

Figure 8–21. Linear amplification with limiting.

often ignored the fact that the typical user of a linear hearing aid would either have to set the gain too low for proper hearing of quiet sounds or else experience excessive loudness over a wide range of sounds in the real world, as illustrated in Figure 8–21.

Figure 8–22 is an attempt to dramatize the fact that limiting is a good solution to a problem that should not be present in the first place. Linear hearing aids unavoidably create a monster, shown here figuratively as the Excessive-Loudness Lion. (The lion was the only animal in the clip art catalog that looked like a monster.) Output limiting is required to tame him, but why did we create him in the first place? The *only* reason for output limiting in hearing aids for Type I loss is because we have *created* this excessive-loudness monster by using *linear* amplifiers that don't have enough intelligence to gradually turn the gain down. Our great prowess in taming him conceals our shame in his creation.

The UCL data of Pascoe argue that even for Type II loss, where some gain is needed for loud sounds, limiting is not required if the proper high-level gain is chosen (Killion & Fikret-Pasa, 1993). Given that most individuals have Type I or Type II hearing loss, we can safely conclude that *output limiting is the wrong approach most of the time.*

Should the Frequency Response Stay Fixed?

Use of fixed-gain linear amplifiers was one error in traditional hearing aid design; use of a fixed frequency response appears to have been anoth-

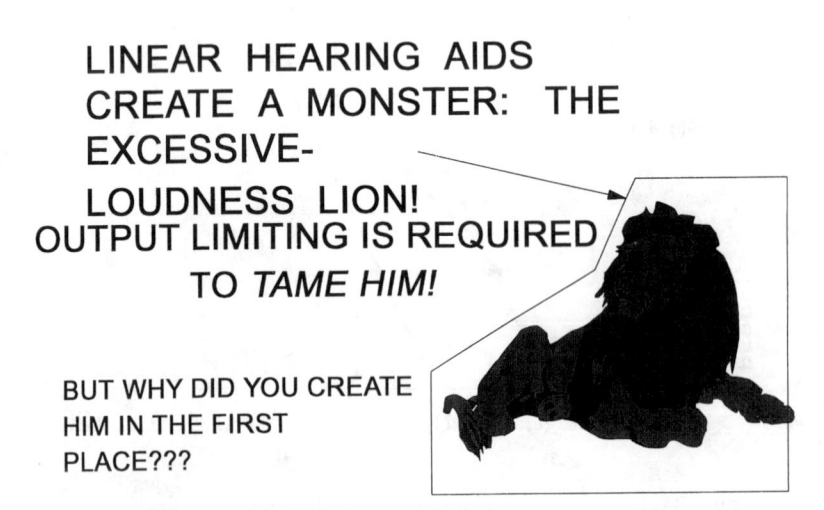

Figure 8–22. Linear Loudness Lion.

er. Most hearing loss is frequency dependent, that is, is greater at some frequencies than others. A 40 dB loss at 1 kHz will more often than not be accompanied by a much greater loss at 4 kHz. Skinner (1976) studied the effect of hearing aid frequency response in her Ph.D. research, using the set of 5 frequency responses shown in Figure 8–23 with subjects having ski-slope hearing loss.

In Figure 8–24, two of Skinner's five frequency responses are shown. The frequency response having the most high-frequency boost (40 dB)

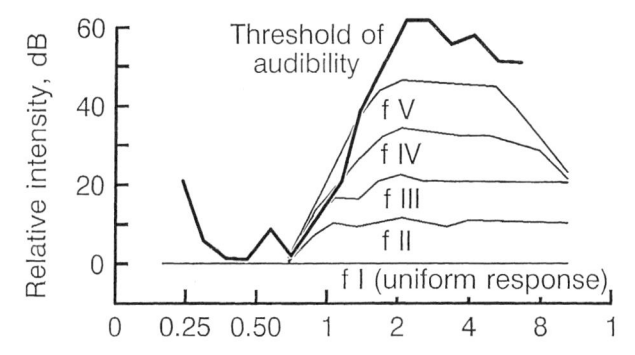

Figure 8–23. Hearing aid frequency responses studied by Skinner using subjects with ski-slope high-frequency losses. (One subject's threshold is shown in dB SPL.)

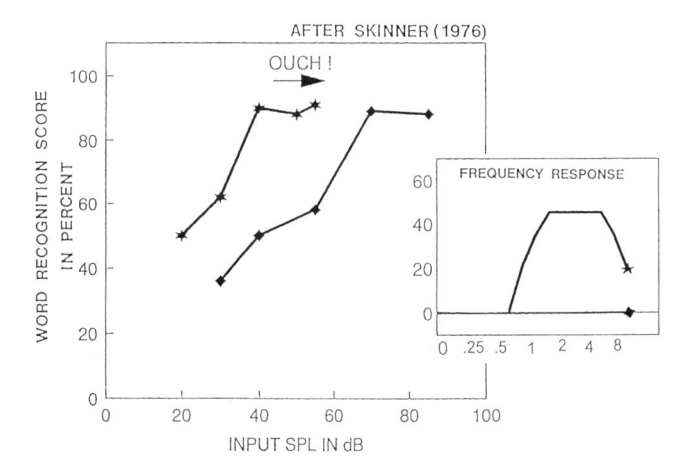

Figure 8–24. Two of Skinner's frequency responses and corresponding intelligibility curves for one of her subjects. (The "Ouch!" is visual shorthand for "exceeds discomfort level").

gave her subjects the best word recognition score for quiet sounds. This should not be surprising, given their high-frequency loss. Although this response gave the best score for low-level inputs, it became intolerable by the time an input of 55 dB SPL was reached (10 dB below conversational speech). At that point, the *output* had reached discomfort. The flat frequency response, on the other hand, gave poor word-recognition scores at low levels, but at high levels it gave scores nearly as good as the best high-frequency-emphasis scores and did not cause discomfort. Intermediate responses (not shown in Figure 8–24) sometimes gave slightly higher maximum scores.

Skinner herself stated the obvious conclusion: It would be a good thing if the frequency response of hearing aids was level dependent. A high-frequency emphasis for quiet sounds and a relatively flat response for loud sounds would represent much better processing than fixed-response linear amplification for most subjects.

Figure 8–25 shows the level-dependent frequency response designed into one single-channel WDRC-TILL amplifier. The acronym TILL was assigned by Killion, Staab, and Preves (1990) to describe hearing aid signal processing which provides "Treble Increases at Low Levels." A commercial two-channel programmable WDRC amplifier can be programmed to provide even greater changes in frequency response with level, changes of the TILL type, suitable for high-frequency hearing loss,

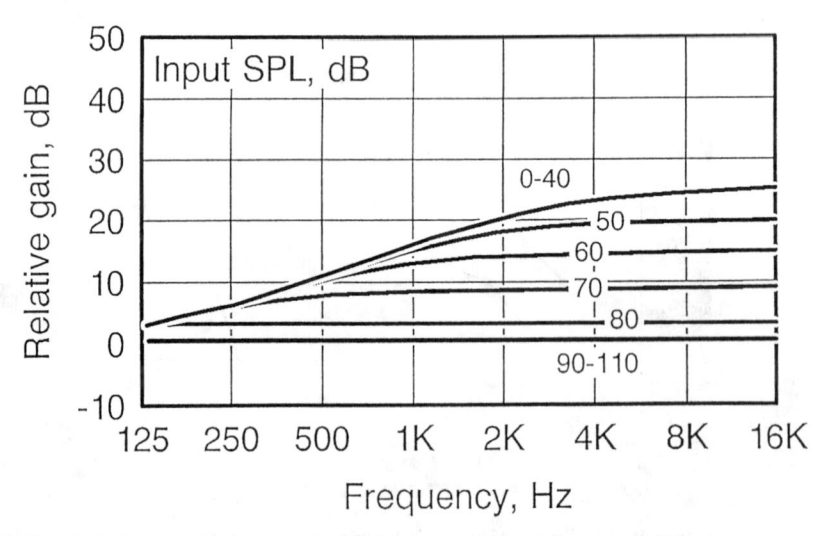

Figure 8–25. Level-dependent frequency response characteristics of commercial WDRC-TILL amplifier.

or of the BILL type (Bass Increases at Low Levels), suitable for reverse-slope loss or for rejecting high-level low-frequency noise.

Leijon (1989) reached a similar conclusion to that of Skinner. Leijon took the Zwicker loudness model, modified it for the widened critical bands typical of moderate-to-severe hearing loss, and calculated the frequency response required of the hearing aid in order to compensate for abnormal loudness perception. Figure 8–26 shows a hearing loss he used as an example, and Figure 8–27 shows the calculated TILL frequency-response set required to compensate for the abnormal loudness corresponding to that loss. Note that we would label the audiogram in Figure 8–26 as having "Type I loss" at low frequencies, but as having "Type II" loss at high frequencies. At high frequencies, therefore, we would expect some loudness loss even for loud sounds. Leijon's calculated required-gain curves shown in Figure 8–27 do indeed show some gain for loud sounds at high frequencies.

Most available WDRC-TILL hearing aid amplifiers can be adjusted to accommodate a Type I loss at low frequencies and a Type II loss at high fre-

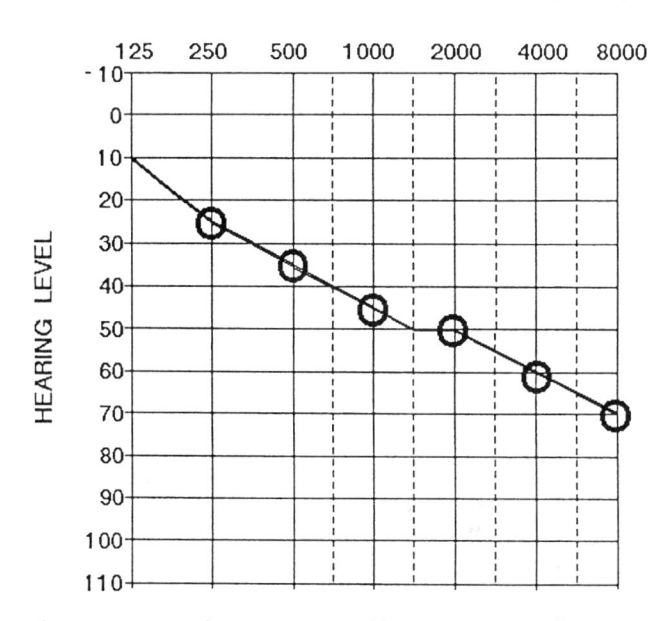

Figure 8–26. Audiogram assumed by Leijon (1991) for Figure 8–27 results.

THEORETICAL INSERTION RESPONSE REQUIRED AT THREE INPUT LEVELS: ADJUSTED LOUDNESS-GROWTH CURVE
(FROM LEIJON, 1991)

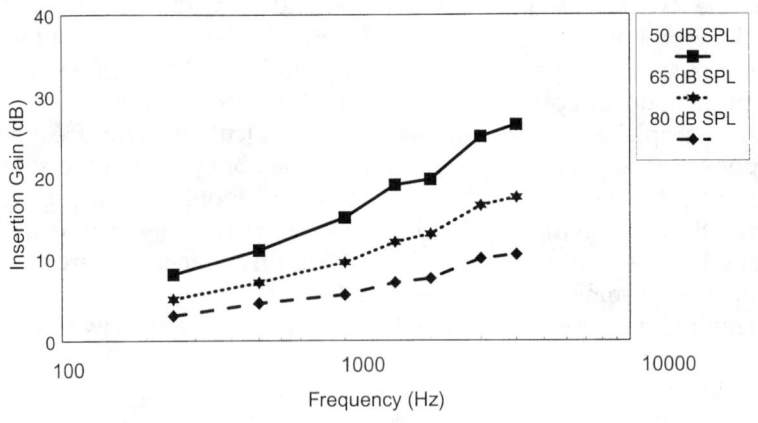

Figure 8–27. Gain-frequency response calculated by Leijon as required to restore normal loudness for hearing loss with Figure 8–26 audiogram.

quencies. Figure 8–28 shows a set of estimated real-ear curves for one such hearing aid, adjusted for someone whose loss progresses from minimal at very low frequencies, through Type I at mid frequencies, to Type II at high frequencies. The curves show 20 dB of gain for loud sounds and 45 dB of gain for quiet sounds at high frequencies, with little or no gain at low frequencies.

Much has been said about the advantages or disadvantages of loudness-based targets. It is certainly true that loudness is not the only important auditory dimension. I believe it is also true, however, that loudness provides the clearest noninvasive picture of the operation and residual capability of the impaired cochlea. Thus, although loudness may not be the final consideration, it appears to many of us to be the best place to start.

Fitting Formulae: FIG6

The need for a systematic approach to fitting the speech sounds into the auditory area has been obvious for years. Fitting formulae of Lybarger, Wallenfels, Burger, Byrne and Dillon (NAL-R), Lyregaard and McCandless (POGO), Cox, Libby, and Seewald (DSL) are currently in use. Several of these are illustrated in Figure 8–29 for a case of high-frequency hearing loss. The pluses represent the NAL-R curve (Byrne & Dillon, 1987), which has received the greatest number of validation studies and is probably the most popular of the formulae suitable for linear hearing aids. A modi-

THEORETICAL INSERTION RESPONSE REQUIRED AT THREE
INPUT LEVELS: ADJUSTED LOUDNESS-GROWTH CURVE
(FROM LEIJON, 1991)

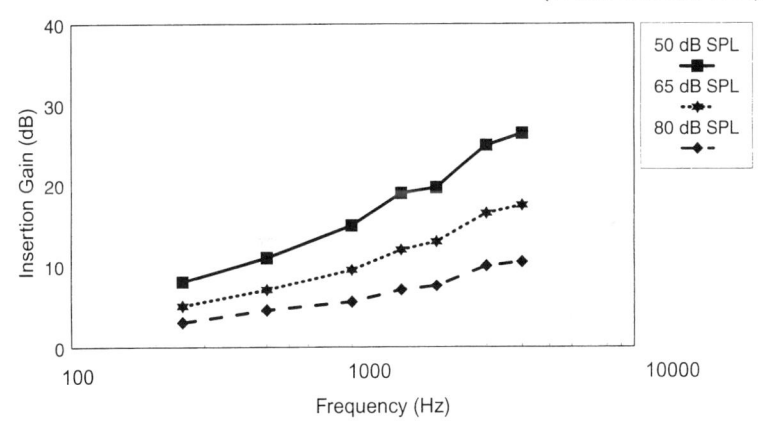

Figure 8–28. Hearing aid showing some gain for high-level sounds at high frequencies, with little gain for high-level sounds at low frequencies, while maintaining basic TILL increase for quiet high-frequency sounds.

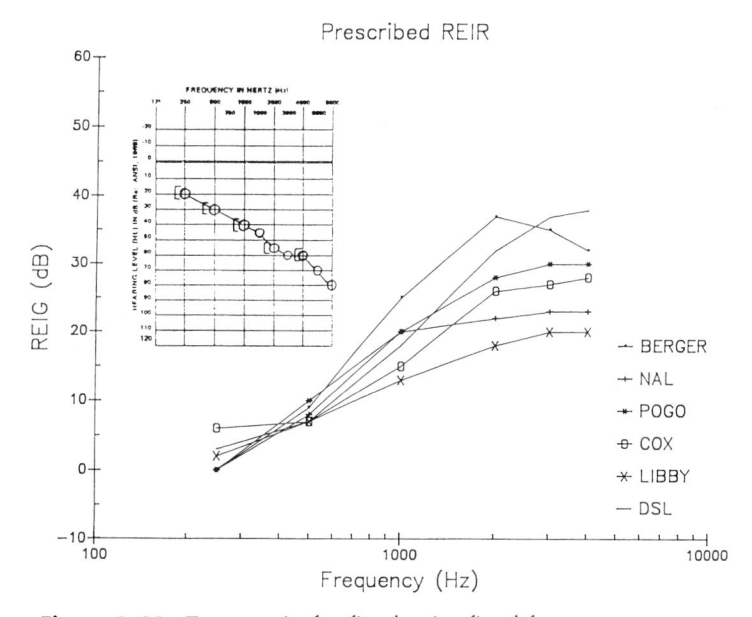

Figure 8–29. Target gain for fixed-gain, fixed-frequency-response hearing aids according to several popular formulae (from Hawkins, Mueller, & Northern, 1992).

fied form of NAL is used by many hearing aid manufacturers when audiologists send in only the impression and an audiogram. I understand that this implicit "you figure it out" request still accompanies the majority of the orders manufacturers receive.

NAL and other targets have served us well, but we need more sophisticated target curves if we wish to move beyond linear, fixed-gain, fixed-response amplification. First and most obvious, one gain and frequency-response target isn't enough if different input levels require different frequency responses.

Various loudness-based fitting methods have been introduced in recent years to provide more sophosticated targets: ELCVIL8, DSL-I/O, P3, and VIOLA. Some use individually-measured loudness data (VIOLA and P3-LGOB), others use audiogram information only, predicting the individual loudness growth from average data (DSL-I/O & P3-Aud+), and some use MCL plus audiometric data to better predict the individual loudness growth from average data (ELCVIL8). The oldest of these appears to be the ELCVIL approach, which was based on Villchur's 1973 and 1987 fitting suggestions.

FIG6, the triple-target method that will be discussed in detail, falls in the audiogram-only class. FIG6 estimates pathologic loudness growth data from published data on loudness growth versus hearing loss. FIG6 gives a set of three fitting targets; for quiet or low-level sounds, conversational sounds, and loud or high-level sounds. The derivation of the loudness-based FIG6 is described in what follows.

The basis for estimating required gain-to-restore-loudness as a function of hearing loss are the data in Figure 8–30, a reproduction of Figure 6 from Killion & Fikret-Pasa (1993). This was an attempt to estimate the hearing aid gain required for different amounts of hearing loss (assuming the loss fell in the Type I and Type II categories):

1. The gain required to restore audibility for low-level (40 dB SPL) sounds;
2. The gain suggested by loudness data for restoring loudness at conversational speech levels (65–70 dB SPL); and
3. The gain required to restore full loudness to intense sounds (85–105 dB SPL). Note: For speech in the sound field, 40, 65, and 95 dB SPL correspond to about 25, 50, and 80 dB HL, respectively.[9]

---

[9]The relationship between 0°-incident speech and SPL is 15 dB, based on the references given in ANSI standard S3.6-1989, resulting in the 50 dB HL equivalence for 65 dB SPL face-to-face speech. In a Northwestern University classroom experiment last year, pairs of students (ages ranging from their 20's to 40's) and their instructor carried on more or less normal two-way conversations at a comfortable conversational distance, with a sound level meter held near the ear of the listener in each case. The range of frequent peak readings was 58 dB to 70 dB, with an average of 64.8 dB. This supports 65 dB SPL (50 HL) as a reasonable choice for the level of typical conversational speech.

TALKING HAIR CELL 161

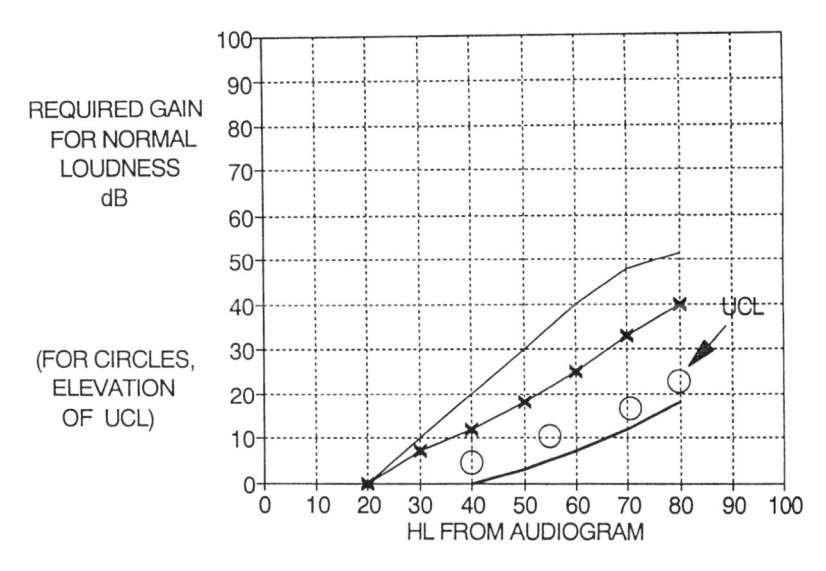

Figure 8–30. Gain required to restore loudness for low-level (———), comfortable-level (X———X), and high-level (———) sounds. UCL data (o) from Pascoe (1988) indicate that the required high-level gain is safe. (Reproduced from Killion & Fikret-Pasa, 1993).

Figure 8–31 shows an example application of the FIG6 procedure. The determination of the three target curves of FIG6 turned out to be fairly straightforward, as explained in the following paragraphs.

1. For quiet sounds, the primary consideration is that of audibility. The hearing aid must provide adequate gain to make quiet sounds audible. At first thought, restoring aided sound-field thresholds to 0 dB HL seems like a good idea in order to restore "normal sensitivity." (Audiologists once thought that way. I can recall Darrell Teter—who was trained at the same university that I was—saying "In those days, baby, if you had a 60 dB loss, I gave you 60 dB of gain!") As discussed by Killion and Studebaker (1978), however, room noise in most locations limits even those with normal hearing to approximately 20 dB masked thresholds.[10] So giving hearing aid wearers sufficient gain to bring their aided sound-field thresholds in a test booth below 20 dB HL will, in most cases, be giv-

---

[10]The Killion and Studebaker paper contains a rule of thumb useful in many situations: Subtract 20 dB from the A-weighted sound level meter reading in a noisy environment and you have a good estimate of the masked sound-field thresholds you could obtain in that environment. Driving 70 mph in many cars produces a 70 dB(A) SPL noise level, for example, so the occupants experience a good simulation of a 50 dB hearing loss. With the most common noise spectra, the masked threshold will be approximately flat from 500 to 4000 Hz.

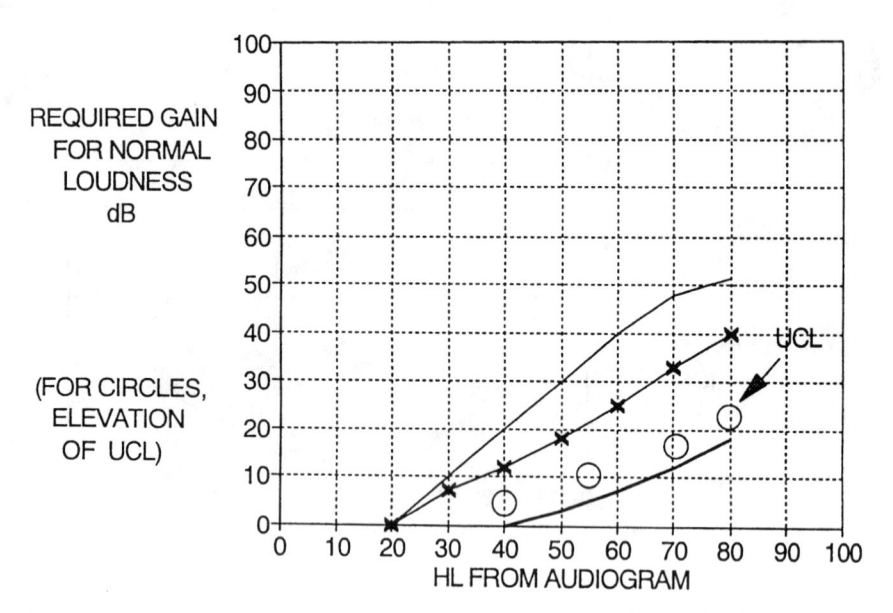

[Figure: plot with y-axis "REQUIRED GAIN FOR NORMAL LOUDNESS dB (FOR CIRCLES, ELEVATION OF UCL)" ranging 0-100, x-axis "HL FROM AUDIOGRAM" 0-100, showing UCL curve with x marks and circles.]

Figure 8–31. FIG6 target gain curves for WDRC hearing aids with level-dependent frequency response. The target curves (and the NAL-R curve) correspond to the audiogram at the top of the figure.

ing them empty (and probably annoying) gain. On the other hand, the quietest elements of conversational speech fall at about 20 dB HL, so *less* gain would leave some conversational speech cues inaudible. The formula for low-level gain thus seemed obvious: G = HL − 20. This is the gain required to produce 20 dB HL sound-field thresholds. No gain is required until the hearing loss exceeds 20 dB. (For losses above 60 dB, some modification is required for practical reasons because of feedback difficulties. A half-gain rule was thus adopted above 60 dB: A gain of 40 dB for a 60 dB loss [60 − 20 = 40], but only 45 dB of gain for a 70 dB loss, 50 dB for 80 dB, etc.). The low-level target shown in Figure 8–31 is labeled "40 dB" meaning 40 dB SPL input.

2. For conversational speech, Pascoe's (1988) data on Most Comfortable Loudness (MCL) as a function of hearing loss were used to estimate required gain. For example, a hearing loss of 60 dB is typically accompanied by an MCL elevation of 24 dB, so 24 dB of gain would be required to restore MCL. The target curve resulting from this application of Pascoe's

data, corresponding to normal 50 dB HL conversational speech,[11] has been labeled "65 dB."

3. For high-level sounds, the required gain was estimated from the loudness-growth data of Lyregaard (1988) and Lippman et al (1977). Their loudness-growth curves for individuals with 40 dB hearing loss became asymptotic to the normal loudness-growth curve at high levels. For individuals with significantly greater hearing loss, the loudness-growth curves also became asymptotic, but not to the normal loudness-growth curve. The curve for a 60-dB loss, for example, appears to approach an imaginary line shifted 8 dB to the right of normal. In their original Figure 6 therefore, Killion & Fikret-Pasa indicate that 8 dB of high-level gain is required for a 60 dB loss, whereas 0 dB of high-level gain is required for a 40 dB loss. Other high-level gain data were estimated in a similar way. The high-level target has been labeled "90 dB" rather than 95 dB because most probe-microphone and test-box equipment will only test up to 90-dB SPL.

The UCL elevation data of Pascoe (1988) were also added to the curves in Killion and Fikret-Pasa's Figure 6 (Figure 8–30 here), with a surprising result: On the average, at least, *the gain required for loud sounds is always less than the elevation in discomfort level*. For example, at 60-dB loss about 8 dB of gain is required for high-level sounds, *but the elevation in UCL is about 12 dB*. Let me say that differently, because it is important. Assume you have a typical 60-dB loss. Your *discomfort* level will be elevated by 12 dB, but you will need only 8 dB of gain in order to experience the same *loudness* for high-level sounds as a person with normal hearing. If you and I sit together at a Chicago hockey game and you wear a hearing aid with 8 dB of gain, by the time the sound level rises to your discomfort level, I will already be 4 dB past my normal-hearing discomfort level. When I first reach discomfort, you will still have a 4 dB margin left before you reach *your* discomfort level.

What the available data and the reasoning of the previous paragraph imply is that we really *have* been doing it wrong all these years. We have been using limiting to cover up our original sin in fitting linear amplifiers. Had we instead used amplifiers that restored loudness sensation to approximately normal, we would not have needed limiting except in

---

[11]Pascoe's data, which show a normal MCL of 60 dB HL, were obtained with pulsed tones. A reasonable single-number approximation to the minimum audible field data is 5 dB SPL (across the audiometric frequencies), so 65 dB SPL would be a reasonable approximation to 60 dB HL. The choice of a slightly different test level will not affect the results significantly with wide-dynamic-range compression hearing aids. (Choosing a 5 dB different level will affect the measured gain only 2.5 dB, for example, if a hearing aid provides 2:1 compression at that test frequency.)

those circumstances where someone with normal hearing would need hearing protection. For those cases, where hearing protection is required, the user of a WDRC aid can simply turn down the volume control.

Based on the deduced gain requirements of the previous figure—and the fact that these are largely independent of frequency as reported by Pascoe (1988) and Lyregaard (1988)—it became a simple matter to fit each of these curves with mathematical formulae. With formulae in hand, can a spreadsheet be far behind?

The FIG6.EXE Computer Spreadsheet

FIG6.EXE is a computer spreadsheet that automatically produces target curves once the audiogram data have been entered. It provides targets for three input levels: 40, 65, and 90 dB SPL. The target curves are plotted to the standard 50 dB/decade hearing-aid scale. This allows ready comparison to measured probe response curves taken at 40 (or 50), 65, and 90 dB SPL. (Hold the measured and calculated curves up to the light and slide them until the scales match; one or the other curve may need to be magnified on a copy machine so both are the same size.) Obtaining the real-ear 40-dB-input curve requires an unusually quiet room and special equipment as of this writing. It is easily checked, however; aided sound-field thresholds should be close to 20 dB HL. (The 40 dB target formula was chosen to produce exactly 20 dB HL aided thresholds.) The NAL-Revised target curve is also displayed by the FIG6 computer program for comparison. Although the NAL-R target is based on an empirical formula and not directly on loudness data, the revised-NAL curve usually lies close to the target curve for 65 dB SPL input except at low frequencies (where NAL always calls for a rolloff) and at 1 kHz (where NAL calls for more gain).

Two cc coupler targets for BTE, ITE, ITC, and CIC hearing aids are available in FIG6, which incorporates the CORFIG data of Killion and Revit (1993). These target response curves can be printed and sent in to the factory if desired.

FIG6.EXE and associated graphical printing software are contained on Band 8 of the enclosed CD. A PrntScrn program is included in the FIG6 disc, so graphs can be printed directly to a LaserJet or Dot matrix printer. Color graphs can be PrntScrn'd to an HP 320® or 500C or 550C Inkjet color printer. The same software package will be sent (on a 3 1/4" disk) gratis to anyone who sends in a self-addressed envelope to Etymotic Research.

Individual loudness growth

The FIG6 program uses average-loudness-based targets. Will these be valid for everybody, or will individual differences be too large to make any average-based approach truly useful? The answer surely lies somewhere in between.

The longstanding success of average-based fitting formulae since Lybarger introduced his famous stored-program fitting computer (a circular slide rule) in 1955 would argue against discarding average-based approaches. On the other hand: (1) loudness tolerance can increase with accommodation to loud sounds, (2) acoustic trauma can produce hypersensitive ears, and (3) some people are simply different.

LDL Shift with Prolonged Exposure

Patients who typically produce aberrant loudness growth judgments include those who have learned to live comfortably with sounds most of us would judge to be uncomfortably loud. Individuals who have accommodated to powerful linear hearing aids will sometimes say WDRC aids are not loud enough.

Figure 8–32 shows interesting loudness accommodation data that came out of an experiment originally aimed at another question: do subjects with hearing impairments judge sound quality in the same way as people with normal hearing, assuming the sound is loud enough to be readily heard by all subjects? Palmer (1994, personal communication)

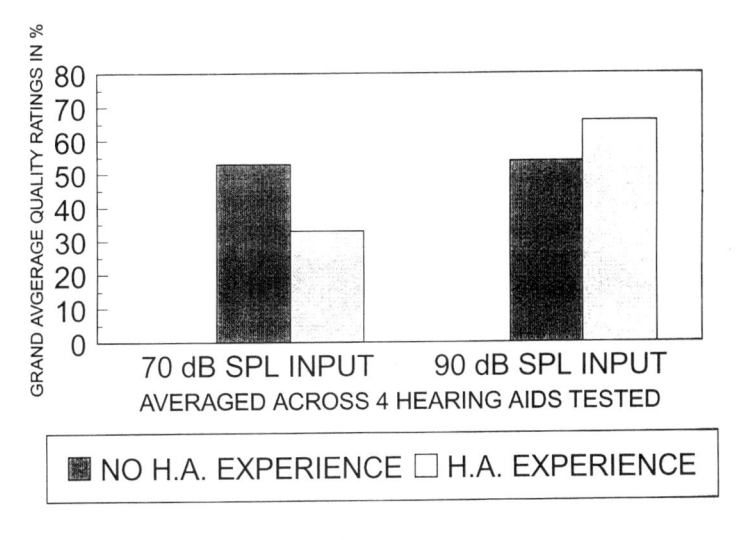

Figure 8–32. Quality judgments for two groups of subjects with hearing impairment. Those experienced in linear hearing aids and those with no hearing aid experience. Note that the experienced users liked it loud!

found an interesting confirmation of the old "Wear it awhile and you'll get used to it" advice. Subjects with hearing impairments who had not been wearing aids judged sound quality in about the same way as people with normal hearing, down-rating the distorted sound of starved Class A hearing aids with 90 dB inputs. Subjects with hearing impairments who had been wearing such hearing aids, on the other hand, didn't mind distortion nearly as much. What they *did* like was *loud*! As shown in Figure 8–32, subjects with no hearing aid experience judged the across-aids average quality for 70 dB and 90 dB inputs about the same. Subjects with hearing aid experience, on the other hand, judged the 70 dB and 90 dB inputs differently: Their across-aid average quality ratings were significantly higher for the louder presentation.

Figure 8–33 shows the shift in loudness function with prolonged exposure to intense industrial noise. These data were obtained roughly 25 years ago in Germany by Niemeyer (1971), who reported that in his measurements, normal-subject loudness discomfort level (LDL) averaged 10 dB above acoustic-reflex threshold (AR), and that the LDL-AR difference did not increase with hearing loss until a very large hearing loss was encountered. At the time, acoustic reflex and loudness discomfort levels

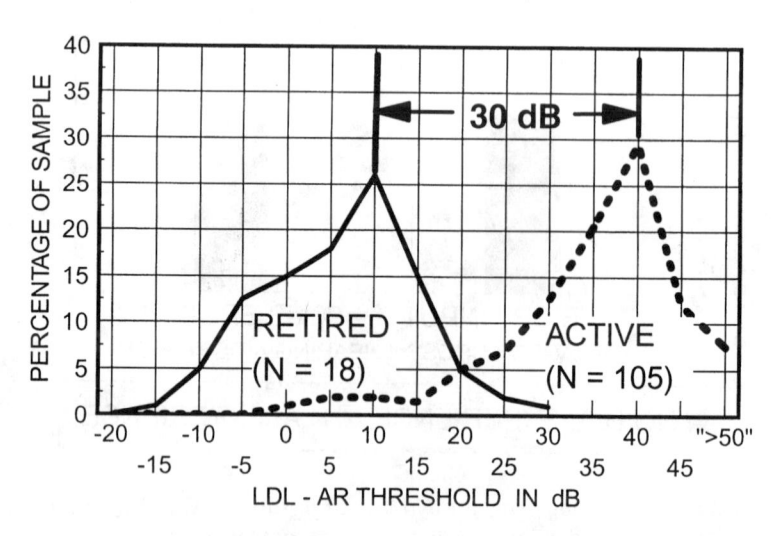

Figure 8–33. Loudness Discomfort Level Shift for workers exposed to intense noise (data of Niemeyer, 1971).

were popular things to compare. More importantly, it was a time when it was possible to find subjects who were still being subjected to intense industrial noise without hearing protection. Niemeyer's surprising finding on some 105 active workers in intense noise was that their LDLs were elevated by 30 dB, exhibiting a typical difference between acoustic reflex and LDL of 40 dB. Loud sounds simply didn't bother these subjects.

The thoughtful thing that Niemeyer did was to double-check his findings not only against individuals with normal hearing but against 18 subjects who had been retired for at least 2 years from working in that same intense-noise environment. When he tested those subjects he found *their LDLs had come back to normal*! So here we see a 30 dB change in LDL from "getting used to it." As he noted, their *hearing* thresholds did not recover, only their LDLs.

When you first fit a hearing aid, it helps to know where the patient's ears have been. I fit my first wife's father with hearing aids when he retired as foreman of a paint plant some 17 years ago, and I couldn't measure his loudness discomfort at the limits of the audiometer. Nothing bothered him. When I fit him with hearing aids, I automatically ordered compression limiting and set the output conservatively, but I did it mostly out of habit; certainly not because I had any LDL problems to worry about. You can perhaps guess the outcome: He retired to Maine where it was quiet, and 2 years later I got a call from him saying, "You know, those hearing aids are a bit uncomfortable [loud] sometimes."

The conclusion appears to be that measurement of individual loudness growth can be valuable in some cases, but any history of high-level noise exposure should be taken into account. Moreover, Knier, and Bentler (1994) reported that approximately 20% of subjects could not reliably perform the loudness task. In cases such as those, the average data provide a good place to start.

PRESENT AND FUTURE PROGRESS

Hearing Aids at High Sound Levels

One of the reasons hearing aids often don't work well is because they distort high-level sounds. Figure 8–34 shows distortion measurements we made recently on three commercial hearing aids: Two Class A hearing aids and one WDRC-TILL hearing aid.

At normal conversational speech levels of 65 dB SPL (frequent peaks on the sound level meter), all three hearing aids operate without distortion. This is true even taking into account the 75 dB SPL instantaneous peaks which accompany 65 dB SPL peak sound level meter (SLM) readings.

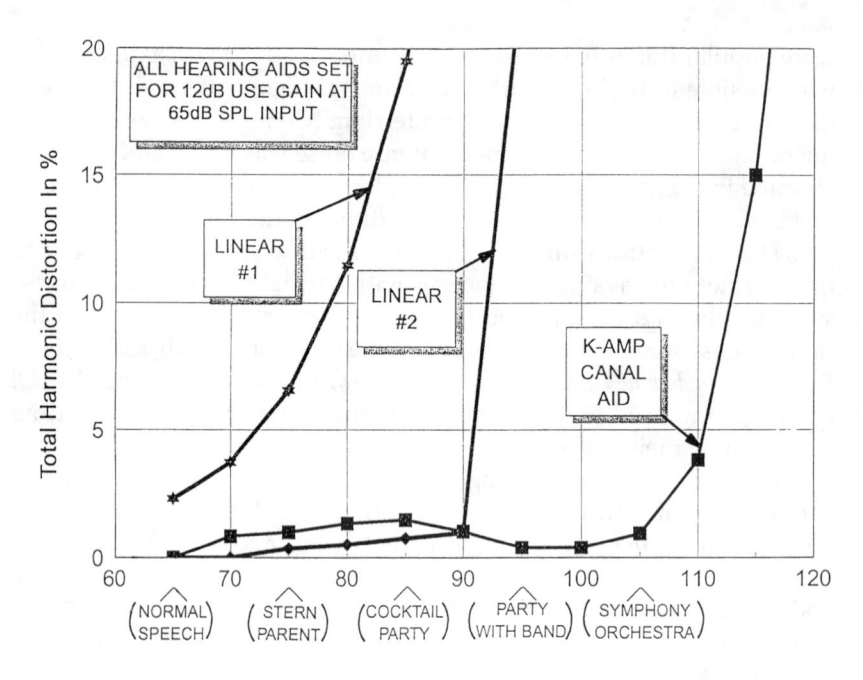

Figure 8–34. Distortion at real-world SPLs for three widely sold hearing aids: two using starved-class-A linear circuits and one using a low-distortion WDRC Class D circuit.

But many circumstances in social situations require low-distortion operation at much higher levels. A raised voice ("stern parent") can easily exceed 75 dB SLM readings. If you take a $32.00 Radio Shack sound level meter with you to parties, you will find that after a few drinks the "cocktail party effect" (Pollack & Pickett, 1957) sets in and the overall SPL rises into the 80s. If a band is playing—whether at a national audiology convention or a Wisconsin farmhouse party—the conversational levels rise into the high 90s. At the two country and western dances where I had a sound level meter, the levels ranged from 100–105 dB SPL.

Although the FDA will not presently permit any benefit claim for reduced hearing-aid distortion (Killion, 1994), it would otherwise seem self-evident that designing hearing aids that can be worn without distortion is a good thing. Distortion erodes intelligibility.

As an amateur violinist, the slide that I most enjoy showing is reproduced in Figure 8–35. As described elsewhere, the violin is a powerful

VIOLINISTS WHO CAN WEAR K-AMP HEARING AIDS WHILE PLAYING:

RUBEN GONZALEZ: CO-CONCERTMASTER, CHICAGO SYMPHONY ORCHESTRA

JOE GOLAN: PRINCIPAL, SECOND VIOLINS, CHICAGO SYMPHONY ORCHESTRA

MILTON PREVES: FORMER PRINCIPAL, VIOLAS, CHICAGO SYMPHONY ORCHESTRA

SAM THAVIU: SOLOIST, NORTHWESTERN UN PROF., FORMER CONCERTMASTER, PITTSBURGH AND CLEVELAND ORCHESTRAS

MEAD KILLION; BUT NO ONE EVER ASKS HIM TO PLAY!

Figure 8–35. Four world-class musicians whose ears attest to the improved performance of modern hearing aids.

instrument, and soloists find their left ears especially at risk (Royster et al., 1991). The sound pressure levels routinely produced by musicians were a major challenge in the design of the hearing aids these musicians can now wear. I am grateful that each of them gave me permission to publish their successful use of these hearing aids.

Acknowledgments: Steve Iseberg, Tim Monroe, Don Wilson, Dennis Ervin, Matt Roberts, and Jonathan Stewart each made a significant contribution to the instrumentation and/or software necessary to provide the "Playing Bach by Ear" recordings of objective Tartini tones. Don Wilson did much of the higher-quality graphics.

REFERENCES

Allen, J. B. (1990). *User manual for the CUB^{e}DIS distortion product measurement system*. AT&T Bell Labs. (Available from Mimosa Acoustics, Box 1111 Mountainside, NJ 07092.)

ANSI (1989). *American National Standard Specification for Audiometers, S3.6-1989.* c/o *Acoustical Soc. Am.*, New York, NY.

Barford, J. (1978). Multichannel compression hearing aids: Experiments and considerations on clinical applicability. *Scandinavian Audiology, 6*, 315–340.

Byrne, D., & Dillon, H. (1986). The National Acoustic Laboratories' (NAL) new procedure for selecting the gain and frequency response of a hearing aid. *Ear and Hearing, 7*, 257–265.

Fikret-Pasa, S. (1993). *The effects of compression ratio on speech intelligibility and quality*. Doctoral dissertation, Northwestern University, Ann Arbor, MI. (University Microfilms.)

Fortune, W. F., Preves, D. A., & Woodruff, B. D. (1991). Saturation-induced distortion and its effects on aided LDL. *Hearing Instruments, 42*(10), 37–42.

French, N. R., & Steinberg, J. C. (1947). Factors governing the intelligibility of speech sounds. *Journal of the Acoustical Society of America, 19*; 90–119.

Goldberg, H. (1966). Hearing aid. U.S. patent no. 3229049 (filed August 4, 1960).

Hawkins, D. B. (1992). Prescriptive approaches to selection of gain and frequency response. In H. G. Mueller, D. B. Hawkins, & J. L. Northern (Eds.), *Probe microphone measurements: Hearing aid selection and assessment* (p. 107, Figure 5–3). San Diego, CA: Singular Publishing.

Hawkins, D. B., Mueller, H. G., & Northern, J. L. (1992) *Probe Microphone Measurements Hearing Aid Selection and Assessment, 107 & 109.*

Hawkins, D. B. & Naidoo, S. V. (1993). A comparison of sound quality and clarity with asymmetrical peak clipping and output-limiting compression. *Journal of the American Academy of Audiology, 4*(4): 221–228.

Hawkins, D. B., Walden, B. E., Montgomery, A., & Prosek, R. A. (1987). Description and validation of an LDL procedure designed to select SSPL90. *Ear and Hearing, 8*(3): 162–169.

Hellman, R. P. (1994). Personal communication.

Hellman, R. P., & Meiselman, C. H. (1990). Loudness relations for individuals and groups in normal and impaired hearing. *Journal of the Acoustical Society of America, 88*(6), 2596–606

Hellman, R. P. and Meiselman, C. H. (1993). Rate of loudness growth for pure tones in normal and impaired hearing. *Journal of the Acoustical Society of America, 93*, 966–975.

Killion, M. C. (1978). Revised estimate of minimum audible pressure: where is the "missing 6dB"? *Journal of the Acoustical Society of America, 63*(5), 1501–1508.

Killion, M. C. (1979). *Design and evaluation of high fidelity hearing aids*. Ph.D. thesis, Northwestern University. Ann Arbor, MI, University Microfilms.

Killion, M. C. (1994a). Why some hearing aids don't work well!! *The Hearing Review, 1*(1): 40–43.

Killion, M. C. (1978). Revised estimate of minimum audible pressure: Where is the "missing 6dB"? *Journal of Acoustical Society of America, 63*(5), 1501–1508.

Killion, M. C. (1979). *Design and evaluation of high fidelity hearing aids.* Ph.D. thesis, Northwestern University. Ann Arbor, MI, University Microfilms.

Killion, M.C. (1994b). The adverse side effects of FDA's hearing aid proscriptions. *Medical Dev. & Diagnost. Ind. 16*(10) 42–48.

Killion, M. C. and Fikret-Pasa, S. (1993). The three types of sensorineural hearing loss: Loudness and intelligibility considerations. *The Hearing Journal, 46*(11): 31–36.

·Killion, M. C. & Revit, L. (1993). CORFIG and GIFROC: Real ear to coupler and back. In G.A. Studebaker, & I., Hochberg (Eds.) *Acoustical factors affecting hearing aid performance* (pp. 65–85). Boston: Allyn & Bacon.

Killion, M. C., Staab, W. J., & Preves, D. A. (1990). Classifying automatic signal processors. *Hearing Instruments, 41*(8): 24–26.

Killion, M. C. & Studebaker, G. A. (1978). A-weighted equivalent of permissible ambient noise during audiometric testing. *Journal of the Acoustical Society of America, 63,* 1633–1635.

Knier, E. C., & Bentler, R. A. (1994). *A clinical procedure for loudness perception measurement.* A poster presentation at the American Academy of Audiology meeting in Richmond, VA.

Leijon, A. (1989). *Optimization of hearing aid gain and frequency response for cochlear hearing losses.* Ph.D. thesis and Chalmers University of Technology Technical Report #189, Goteborg, Sweden.

Lippman, P. R., Braida, L.D., & Durlach, N. I. (1978). New results on multiband amplitude compression for the hearing impaired. *Journal of the Acoustical Society of America, 62:*590(A).

Lybarger, S. (1955). Basic manual for fitting Radioear hearing aids. Pittsburgh, Radioear Corporation.

Lyregard, P. E. (1988). POGO and the theory behind. In J. Jensen, (Ed.): *Hearing Aid Fitting: Theoretical and Practical Views.* Proceedings of the 13th Danavox Symposium, Copenhagen: 81–94.

Niemeyer, W. (1971). Relations between the discomfort level and the reflex threshold of the middle ear muscles. *Audiology, 10*: 172–176.

Palmer, C. V. (1994). Personal communication.

Pascoe, D. L. (1988). Clinical measurements of the auditory dynamic range and their relation to formulas for hearing aid gain. In J. Jensen, (Ed.), *Hearing aid fitting: Theoretical and practical views.* (pp. 129–152). Proceedings of the 13th Danavox Symposium, Copenhagen.

Pollack, I., & Pickett, J. M. (1957). Cocktail party effect. *Journal of the Acoustical Society of America, 29,* 1328–1329.

Royster, J. D., Royster, L. H., & Killion, M. C. (1991). Sound exposures and hearing thresholds of symphony orchestra musicians. *Journal of the Acoustical Society of America, 89,* 2793–2803.

Ruggero, M. A., & Rich, N. C. (1991). Furosemide alters organ of Corti mechanics: Evidence for feedback of outer hair cells upon the basilar membrane. *Journal of Neuroscience, 11,* 1057–1067.

Skinner, M. W. (1976). Speech intelligibility in noise-induced hearing loss: Effects of high frequency compensation. Doctoral dissertation, Washington University, Ann Arbor, MI. (University Microfilms)

Steinberg, J. C., & Gardener, M. B. (1937). The dependence of hearing impairment on sound intensity. *Journal of the Acoustical Society of America, 9*, 11–23.

Villchur, E. (1973). Signal processing to improve speech intelligibility in perceptive deafness. *Journal of the Acoustical Society of America 53*, 1646–1657.

Villchur E. (1987). Multichannel compression processing for profound deafness, *Journal of Rehabilitation Research and Development 24*(4) 135–148.

Villchur, E. (1993). A different approach to the noise problem of the hearing impaired. In J. Berlin & G. R. Jensen (Eds.), *Recent Developments in Hearing Aid Technology*. Proceedings of the 15th Danavox Symposium, Danavox Jubilee Foundation (Taastrup, DENMARK): 69–80.

Waldhauer, F., & Villchur, E. (1988). Full dynamic range multiband compression in a hearing aid. *The Hearing Journal, 41*(9): 29–31.

INDEX

A

Acadians, 88–92
Acetylcholine, 32–46, 80
Adenosine triphosphate, 46–47
Amplitude compression, 114–118
　1970s–1980s research, 122–123
Antibiotics, 74
　hair cell responses to, 81–82
Audiograms, 99, 100, 102–106, 107, 108, 135
Auditory brainstem responses, 100, 101, 107, 108

C

Charcot-Marie-Tooth syndrome, 101, 107
Children, sensorineural hearing impairment in, 87
Cochlea,
　efferent innervation, 32–32
　function, 29–32, 110
　operation of, 135–137
Cochlear outer hair cells, 73
　electrical properties, 78–80
　function, 77–78
　morphology, 74–77. *See also*: Outer hair cells.
Compression. *See* Amplitude compression.
Cubic distortion product tone, 126

D

Deafness mouse, 93–95
Deiter's cells, 12–14, 21–22, 31
dn gene, 87, 93–94
DNA linkage analysis, 89–92, 94–96
Drugs. *See* Pharmacologic agents.

E

Efferent innervation of hair cells, 80–81
Electromotility of outer hair cells, 3–4, 6–7
　cell turgor, 17–21
　energy sources, 7–12
　volume changes, 19–21

F

FIG6 fitting formula, 158–163
　FIG6.EXE computer spreadsheet, 164–165
Frequency responses, and hearing aids, 154–158

173

G

Genetics, and hearing impairment, 87, 94–95
   deafness, mutant mouse, 93–95
   Usher syndrome, 88–92
Gentamicin, 74, 81–82

H

Hair cells, 73–74
   antibiotics ototoxic effects, 74, 81–82
   efferent innervation of, 80–81
   electrical properties, 78–80
   function, 77–78
   loss of, 87
   morphology, 74–77. *See also* Inner hair cells and Outer hair cells.
Hearing aids, 99, 106–107, 108, 110, 125
   amplitude compression, 114–118, 122–123
   different hearing loss types requirements, 144–147
   FIG6 fitting procedure, 158–163
   fixed frequency response, 154–158
   music and, 134–135, 137–138, 168–169
   noise suppression, 118–121
   outer hair cells and, 108–110
   output limiting, 152–154
   recruitment, 113–114, 123
   sound distortion and, 167–168
   wide-dynamic-range-compression, 150–154
Hearing loss,
   neural versus outer hair cell, 99–101
   types of, 142–144
Hydraulic skeleton concept, 4, 16–17

I

Inner ear, 4
   Bekesy's research, 4–5
   mechanoreceptors, 73
   pharmacologic agents application, 82–84
Inner hair cells,
   cochlea operation, 135–137
   hearing loss and, 101

K

Kresge Hearing Research Laboratory, ix–x

L

Loudness growth data, 137–142

M

Mouse,
   deafness, mutant, 93–95
   hearing impairment in, 88
Music,
   hearing aid requirements, 145–146, 151–152, 168–169
   Tartini tone, 125–128

N

NAL-R curve, 140
Neural hearing loss, 99, 110
Neurotransmitters, in outer hair cells, 32–48, 52
   acetylcholine, 32–46
   adenosine triphosphate, 46–47
   GABA, 47, 49
   receptor mechanisms, 49–52
Noise suppression, in hearing aids, 118–121

O

Olivocochlear nerve bundle, 31–32
Organ of Corti, 6, 9, 29, 87, 93
   architectonics of, 12–14, 21–22
Otoacoustic emissions, 4, 5, 57, 125
   evoked, 57–62

INDEX   175

outer hair cell involvement, 5–6
spontaneous, 57–58
suppression characteristics, 62–66
suppression studies, 59–62
Outer hair cells,
chemical interactions, 29
cochlea operation, 135–137
distortion products, 133–134
electromotility of, 3–4, 6–7
energy sources, 7–12
hydraulic skeleton concept, 4, 16–17
intracellular domains, 14–16
mechanical function, 6–7, 29–32
neurotransmitters, 32–48
organ of Corti structure, 12–14
otoacoustic emissions involvement, 5–6
receptor mechanisms, 49–52
turgor, 17–21
volume changes, 19–21
Outer hair cells hearing loss,
characteristics, 99–101
hearing aids and, 108–110

P

Pharmacologic agents, inner ear application, 82–84
Polymerase Chain Reaction (PCR), 89, 96

R

Recruitment, 113–114, 123
physiological basis, 118

S

Semicircular canal type II hair cells, 73
electrical properties, 78–80
function, 77–78
morphology, 74–77
Spiral ganglion hearing loss, 101
Speech amplification, 114–117
Streptomycin, 74, 81–82
Suppression of otoacoustic emissions, 59, 70, 101, 106, 110
binaural, 66–70
characteristics, 62–66
contralateral, 66–70
ipsilateral, 66–70
noise duration effect, 68–70
studies of, 59–62

T

Tartini tone, 125–128
Transient evoked otoacoustic emissions, 59, 66–70
suppression characteristics, 62–66
suppression studies, 59–62
Type I hearing loss, 142–143
hearing aid requirements, 144–145, 146, 147
output limiting and, 153–154
Type II hearing loss, 143–144
hearing aid requirements, 145–146
output limiting and, 153–154
Type III hearing loss, 144–145
hearing aid requirements, 144–145

U

Usher syndrome, 87, 88–92
Acadians and, 88–92

W

Wen Kresge Echomaster Program, 102, 106
Wide-dynamic-range-compression hearing aids, 150–154
amplifiers, 150–151

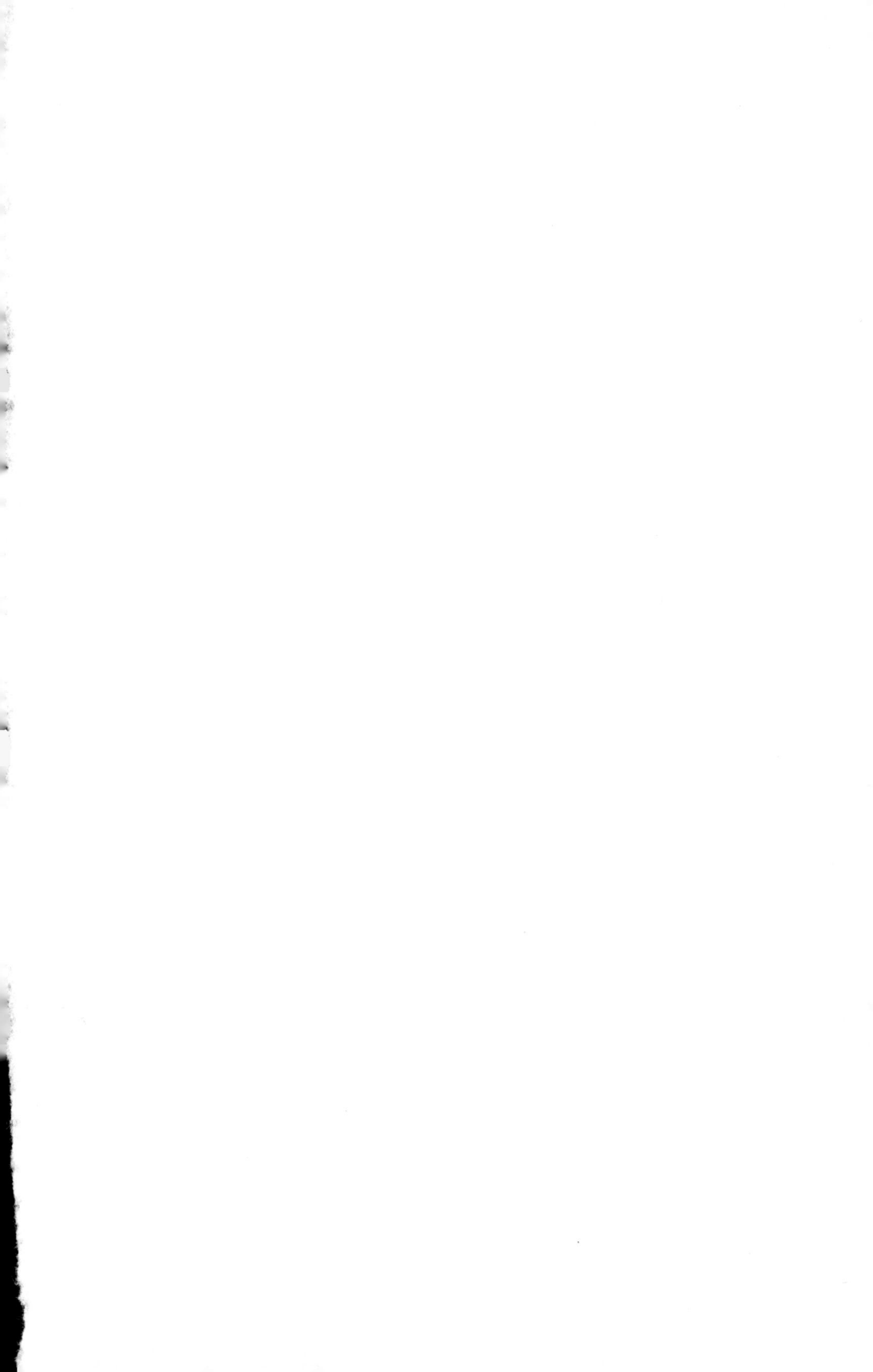